Caring and Nursing: Explorations in Feminist Perspectives

Ruth M. Neil and Robin Watts, Editors

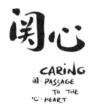

CARING
闭 PASSAGE
TO THE
'心' HEART

Center for Human Caring

National League for Nursing • New York
Pub. No. 14-2369

This book was set in Goudy by Publications Development Company. The editor and designer was Allan Graubard. Clarkwood Corporation was the printer and binder. The cover was designed by Lillian Welsh.

Manufactured in the United States of America.

About the Authors

Elizabeth R. Berrey, PhD, RNCS, is Associate Clinical Professor, Frances Payne Bolton School of Nursing, Case Western Reserve University, Cleveland, Ohio, and Director of Residential Treatment, Bellefaire/Jewish Children's Bureau, University Heights, Ohio.

Elise Boulding, PhD, is Professor Emerita, Dartmouth College, Hanover, New Hampshire.

Margaret A. Crowley, MS, RN, is Staff Nurse, Gero-Psychiatric Unit, Elliot Hospital, Manchester, New Hampshire, and Doctoral Student, University of Texas, Austin, Texas.

Mary E. Duffy, PhD, RN, is Associate Professor, College of Nursing, University of Utah, Salt Lake City, Utah.

Delores A. Gaut, PhD, RN, is Visiting Professor, University of Portland, Portland, Oregon.

Barbara Hedin, PhD, RN, is Clinical Staff Nurse, Oncology/Hospice, The Retreat Hospital, Richmond, Virginia.

Carol Green-Hernandez, PhD, RNC, FNS, is Associate Professor of Nursing, School of Nursing, University of Vermont, Burlington, Vermont.

Sharon Horner, MSN, RN, is PhD Candidate in the Nursing Program, Medical College of Georgia, Athens, Georgia.

Peggy Keen, MS, RN, works in the Infectuous Disease Clinic, Grady Memorial Hospital, Atlanta, Georgia, and is a PhD Candidate in Nursing, Georgia State University, Atlanta, Georgia.

Nina A. Klebanoff, MSN, RNCS, is in independent practice, Dallas Geriatric Services and is a Home Health Care Clinical Specialist. She is also a PhD Candidate at Texas Women's University, Denton, Texas.

Virginia Knowlden, EdD, RN, is Associate Professor and Director of the Master's in Nursing Program, Psychiatric-Mental Health Nursing, Division of Nursing, St. Joseph College, West Hartford, Connecticut.

Kathleen I. MacPherson, PhD, is Professor and Associate Dean, School of Nursing, University of Southern Maine, Portland, Maine.

Karen L. Miller, PhD, RN, is Assistant Director of Nursing/ Administrative Research, The Children's Hospital, and Assistant Professor, School of Nursing, University of Colorado Health Sciences Center, Denver, Colorado.

Ruth M. Neil, MN, RN, is PhD Candidate, University of Colorado Health Sciences Center, Denver, Colorado.

Susan Poslusny, MSN, RN, is PhD Candidate, College of Nursing, University of Illinois, Chicago, Illinois.

Carol Roberts, MSN, RN, is Associate Professor of Nursing, University of New Hampshire, Durham, New Hampshire.

Sheila K. Smith, MSN, RN, is Instructor/Lecturer, School of Nursing, University of Wisconsin, Eau Claire, Wisconsin.

Debbie Ward, PhD, RN.

Robin Watts, MSN, RN, is PhD Candidate, University of Colorado Health Sciences Center, Denver, Colorado.

Denise Webster, PhD, RNCS, is Associate Professor, School of Nursing, University of Colorado, Denver, Colorado.

Marylouise Welch, PhD, RN, is Assistant Professor, St. Joseph College, West Hartford, Connecticut.

Patricia Yaros, PhD, RN.

Contents

Preface

This work is an official publication of the Center for Human Caring. It is an outgrowth of the National Conference on Caring and Nursing: Explorations in Feminist Perspectives, organized by the Doctoral Student Group at the University of Colorado School of Nursing/Center for Human Caring, and held there in June 1988. Special recognition for organization and editing this important work is given to Ruth Neil and Robin Watts, both PhD candidates at the University of Colorado School of Nursing.

Because the publication of this work is an official activity of the Center for Human Caring, it is consistent with the Center's goals and activities. The Center for Human Caring is exploring new ways to advance the art and science of human caring in education, research, and practice. The efforts in the Center range from curriculum work to developing new philosophies, theories, and methods associated with the knowledge of caring.

To my knowledge, this conference on nursing and caring in the feminist perspective was the first of its kind. It attracted nurses and colleagues from other disciplines to elucidate the conflicts, oppression, challenges, and issues associated with connections and commonalities between feminist perspectives and caring in nursing.

As noted in my earlier work (1990), "It is perhaps not coincidental that feminism and nursing are increasingly linked in the literature. Nursing, women, and children are perhaps the paradigm cases for 'invisible' care value issues and help us understand why caring values are not core for health care policy and practice" (p. 63).

We are all now aware that the present health care system operates within a patriarchal structure and caring is not valued because it is viewed as women's work. We also know that caring is linked to the survival of humanity and so is a caring feminist perspective linked to a morality that will help to preserve civilization against the annihilation of all living things. Caring and the feminist lens that nursing can use to uncover, examine, reclaim, and restore itself is the antidote now called for in the non-caring, bureaucratic health care system. The chaos of the present patriarchal model must now yield to moral ideals of caring and make room for a caring feminist model that nursing brings to the health and healing processes of life. As this occurs, our future system will give way to more women and nurses as healers and empowered leaders, resulting in a new force.

This special conference provided public space for the awakening of nursing to its solid soul connection with caring and feminist views. This Center for Human Caring publication serves as a means for the further awakening of more nurses, and colleagues in other disciplines.

My thanks and continuing appreciation go to the National League for Nursing for being a partner with the Center for Human Caring and in helping to create continuous clearings for the new possibilities for nursing and the health sciences, and by agreeing to be the official publication outlet for Center for Human Caring projects and activities.

Jean Watson
Dean and Professor
School of Nursing
University of Colorado Health Sciences Center
Boulder, CO

REFERENCES

Watson, J. (1990). The moral failure of the patriarchy. *Nursing Outlook, 38*(2), 62–66.

Introduction

The papers included in this publication were presented in 1988 at a conference organized and sponsored by the Doctoral Student Group and the Center for Human Caring at the University of Colorado Health Sciences Center School of Nursing. The conference was born out of an informal lunchtime conversation among a group of students interested in the impact of feminist scholarship on the development of nursing knowledge. The inherent connections between feminist perspectives and caring seemed apparent. From this discussion came the query as to how nurse scholars around the country were exploring and developing these connections. In the belief that many other nurses were probably seeking answers to similar questions, a commitment was made to organize an opportunity for nurses involved in developing and applying knowledge in these areas to share with their colleagues. Apparently, the "time was right." Planning committee members were gratified with the response to the call for abstracts and with the quality of the papers that were ultimately presented.

The organizing committee is delighted with this new opportunity to share the contents of the conference with a far wider audience. Although the current authors are receiving recognition for "conference-organizing success," by virtue of this publication, this recognition must also be shared with several colleagues in the Doctoral Program at the University of Colorado. Especially to be mentioned are Linda Bergstrom, Nancy Case, Roxie Foster, Karen Kristensen, Leslie Skillman, Judy Igoe, Fran Reeder, Jura Sakalys, and Denny Webster.

The purpose of this Introductory Chapter is to "whet the appetites" of potential readers of this publication. Although reference is made to specific comments by several of the presenters, we have not made an effort to cite

1

exact page numbers where those comments appear. In part, this is to stimulate you, the reader, to read the entire work cited.

We wish the readers could experience the sense of warmth, support, and inspiration that prevailed during the two days of sharing. Perhaps this enthusiastic introduction, and the obvious credibility of the proceeding papers, will convey some of that "wonderfully remembered" feeling. The very positive atmosphere was generated not only by the high caliber of papers presented, but also by the willingness to share and participate on the part of all who attended. There was both harmony and debate on a scholarly level, but there was no dissonance in personal relationships. As Nina Klebanoff pointed out, feminism embraces diversity and interconnection. The theme of the conference became a lived experience. This experience was mirrored in Susan Poslusny's paper in which she defined friendship as "an experience shared by individuals that creates a climate of discovery, encourages learning about oneself and about others, and creates shared meaning about the world and reality." Many lasting friendships emerged from the conference.

For some, if not many, of the participants, the conference was an important milestone marking personal and cognitive growth, of "finding their voice," to use the terminology of Belenky et al. (1986). From experiencing life "in silence" through listening to and parroting others' voices and opinions, to having the knowledge and confidence to express one's own knowing and experience in language that is understandable to others is a valid way to describe the feminist experience, and the nursing experience. It was evident to all present the contributors were living out their personal commitments regarding what is important in their lives and in the world. They were the kind of people who, in the words of Margaret Farley (1986), ". . . allow us grounds for counting on one another (because of their commitments and scholarship . . .) . . . the chaotic uncertainty of the future is contained in the faculty to make and keep promises" (p. 19).

That this personal and scholarly commitment is still being enacted two years following the conference is evident from the continuing contributions of those who participated. Their contributions in their workplaces, communities, or through other publications can be documented for nearly all contributors. A stellar example is Dr. Elise Boulding, a keynote speaker for the conference, who was nominated in 1989 for a Nobel Peace Award.

The pervasive tone of the conference was positive. In the words of Sheila Smith, we were "doing feminism" with the emphasis, as Elise Boulding described it, on being "shapers," not victims. A number of the presentors focused on raising consciousness, or provided timely reminders of behaviors that act as barriers or negate nurses' potential "shaping role" in the health care system. Peggy Keen's *Oppression Checklist* is a most useful aid in this regard. As Peggy pointed out, the purpose of the checklist is to bring "unconscious behaviors out of the closet so that we can examine them in the light of day—see what may be happening, and change the behaviors that ultimately are 'uncaring'." As Friere has stated, it is vital to reveal the world of oppression without illusion in order to transcend it. Carol Roberts presented an excellent example of this by raising the question of whether horizontal violence occurs in nurses toward mothers of the chronically mentally ill patients they care for.

In keeping with Friere's wisdom, other presentors drew our attention to dominating and institutionalized power relations that stubbornly resist attempts to implement change. The theme from Kathleen MacPhersons's keynote paper was that the influence of the social context in which nurses practice (and the inherent power relations and dominant values) must be transformed. This theme was reiterated throughout the conference. Two years after the conference, in 1990, these challenges remain. An ever increasing budget deficit in the United States, with cost-cutting in social services being the only acceptable political solution to offer, adoption of economic rationalism as the dominant economic paradigm in Australia, political solutions which further widen the gap between the "haves" and the "have-nots" in Britain, all indicate a worsening social context for various national health care systems whose primary concern(s) should be the welfare of people.

If nursing and nurses are to meet these challenges and play a decisive role in the transformation and reshaping of our present illness care system—and the achievement of a more just allocation of resources—a number of changes, both personal and professional, must occur. Those of us who have not already done so will need to adopt a new perspective on feminine qualities and values. Elise Boulding's example of styles of nurturance is a case in point: nurturing roles "which are at the same time autonomous and self-respecting, as distinct from earlier styles of subservient nurturance." We will need to further develop and strengthen the embryonic sense of community and colleagueship among nurses and initiate or augment local, national, and international networks. As Patricia Yaros indicated, the lack of unity within nursing is an obvious stumbling block to the achievement of an equitable, caring system.

We must be actively involved in defining our own reality, not passively accepting a reality defined for us by others. As Denise Webster pointed out, ". . . we need to name our experiences using our own voices and be actively involved in creating and communicating our own definitions of our values . . ." (If we can achieve this while still retaining our sense of humor, as Denise has obviously managed to do, we will definitely be "ahead of the game.") This activity would assist in reversing the themes of invisibility and marginality identified in Karen Miller's study. Sheila Smith's feminist analysis of the constructs of health represents another contribution to this renaming of experience.

We need to dialogue, in the true sense of the word, with each other and with those for whom we are caring. Margaret Crowley stressed this in her discussion on nurturing the ethical ideal in nursing. "We must seek to create a caring dialogue with our students that will foster their ability to make moral choices under conditions of oppression, choices that enhance rather than diminish their vision of themselves as caring practitioners." This theme emerged again in Virginia Knowlden's and Carol Hernandez's studies of caring in nursing and nurses, and Sharon Horner's caring model focusing on intersubjective copresence.

We must value our history and celebrate those nurses from whose experiences we can learn. A reconstruction of that history through a feminist lens will also undoubtably provide us with many more valuable lessons and guides. As Elizabeth Berry so proudly affirmed, ". . . we come from a long line of women of courage—our foresisters in nursing." On the other hand, both Elizabeth's paper and Marylouise Welsch's analysis of Florence Nightingale (in the context of 19th-century England) highlighted aspects of our history which have been negative, for us as women and as nurses, that we need to transform.

All this entails hard work. As Debbie Ward so succinctly put it, "Caring *is* work!" and "Nursing . . . is at work on determining the stuff of caring." Barbara Hedin and Mary Duffy echoed this theme in their summary when they indicated that feminist methodology in nursing research, as in the field of sociology, was in the process of becoming. "There is much yet to be explored, created, and envisioned as we open our minds to new paradigms."

It is to that exploration, dialogue, creativity, vision, and associated action that this collection of papers is dedicated. We hope that the ideas contained herein will inspire other nurses to embrace the ideals of caring and adopt the values and approaches foundational to the feminist perspective. Both decisions/actions will contribute to the kind of human relationships needed to make this world a more peaceful, humane, and healthy planet.

Ruth M. Neil, MN, RN, PhD Candidate
University of Colorado

Robin Watts, MSN, RN, PhD Candidate
University of Colorado

REFERENCES

Belenky, M. F., Clinchy, B. M., Goldgerger, N. R., & Tarule, J. M. (1986). *Women's ways of knowing.* New York: Basic Books, Inc.

Farley, M. A. (1985). *Personal commitments: Making, keeping, breaking.* New York: Haper & Row.

1

Caring and Nursing: Explorations in Feminist Perspectives — Introductory Remarks

Delores A. Gaut

As I reflected on these introductory remarks, I glanced at the conference program and saw an obvious title—*Caring and Nursing: Explorations in Feminist Perspectives*. Because those three concepts have received much of my attention over the last several years, it seems appropriate that I address caring, nursing, and feminism briefly.

When I speak of caring, I am speaking of a distinct way of thinking, believing, and acting that calls for commitment and hard choices. When I speak of a life of caring, I am speaking of a life committed to helping others grow and actualize themselves. Caring is not merely liking, or comforting, or wishing others well; rather, caring is a stance of respect for all living things that requires knowledge, trust, hope, honesty, and courage.

Lucy of Peanuts fame once said. "I can love humanity, it's people I can't stand." Lucy exemplifies a common human attitude, for it is easier to speak of caring in the great abstract than it is to deal with concrete situations in everyday life.

Caring does not involve projection into another person, nor does it imply full understanding of the other person. Caring involves receiving an "other" in a responsive and receptive manner. If you define yourself as a caring person, then your responsibility is to develop your capacity to experience the other person and be receptive to that person's needs. Caring is a natural way to relate to another human being, and in that relating, both persons become more human.

The notion that caring is the essence of nursing, or at the very least an ethical injunction for professional nursing practice, has been written about, researched, and discussed with renewed interest, clarity, and a sense of urgency among nurses and other helping professionals. Science and technology, of course, have had a major impact on the process and acts of caring within illness care institutions. In addition to this impact, one must ask if the individuals providing care adhere to either a professional or a personal value such as caring as a standard for their actions.

To accept caring as a professional value provides a normative standard to govern nursing's actions and attitudes toward those for whom we care. To accept caring as a moral value is to accept the responsibility to improve the welfare of all human beings. Morality not only governs the relations of persons one to one, but also serves as a social conscience that is greater than personal needs. The absence of caring from the current institutional scene is neither individual failure nor casual accident; it is the inevitable consequence of what we as a society and a government have explicitly sought out as the articulating spirit of these institutions.

To accept caring as both a professional and personal value is of central importance not only to the future of nursing as a profession, but to the future of health and illness care in this society.

I suggest that one's commitment to caring is also quite similar to one's commitment to feminism. Nonetheless, both terms are misunderstood, misrepresented, and frequently argued about.

A commitment to feminism is a commitment to the dignity, humanity, and equality of all human beings, which leads to structural changes that occur to the equal good of all. A personal commitment to feminism and to caring as a standard for professional nursing practice can only lead to the demand for major changes in the structure and provision of health care service to all human beings.

It is a major premise of feminism and caring that the process of development is just as important as the product developed. As we review the numbers of participants and presenters at this conference, there is little question of the level of product excellence. The "lived experience" of this conference will answer the question of process and personal development as the truth of each person present is recognized and affirmed.

Throughout this conference I encourage you to remember who you are, where you have been, and where you are going. Each one of us, through the process of discovering, claiming, and acting on the deepest truths of our experience, will free ourselves, and in doing so will recognize we are all part of one another.

2

How Women Are Reshaping Community, Locally and Globally

Elise Boulding

When discussing the reshaping of community, I am referring, of course, to the context for the work of healing. When current social structures are faulty, social values corrupt, and spiritual values absent, the work of healing cannot take place as it should. Underlying the faulty structures of our fragmented society is a pervasive absence of women in shaping roles. Women are assigned to isolated niches where they are supposed to do their work. The isolation of the woman healer from the larger enterprise of healing in our world, and from the governance which should see to the wise allocation of resources for the meeting of human needs, is part of the general victimage of women.

ARE WOMEN VICTIMS OR SHAPERS?

It is too easy, however, to give way to a victim mentality and thus fail to see the ways in which women, despite the difficulties already mentioned, are changing the very world which has for so long constrained them. In this regard, I offer two contrasting pictures of the situation of woman in the world. Figure 1 depicts the forces that oppress her. Woman stands imprisoned inside the tight

Figure 1
The Agents of Oppression for Women*

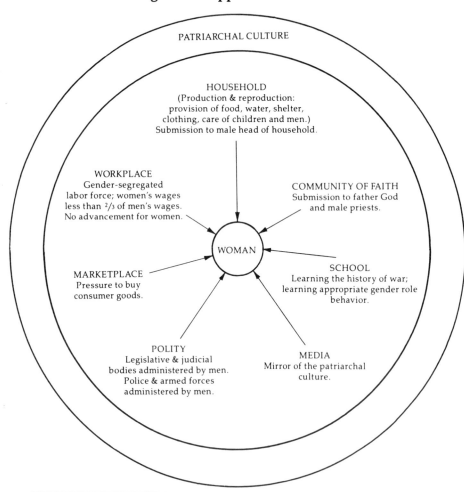

* From Womens Movements and Social Transformation in the Twentieth Century, E. Boulding, in The
Changing Structure of World Politics, Y. Sakamoto, ed., Wanami Shoten Publishers, Tokyo, Japan,
1988.

circle of a patriarchal culture whose institutions ensure her victimization. In
the household, she carries the burden of production and reproduction as she
serves the needs of children and men, always in the context of obedience to
the male head of household. In the community of faith, she is to submit her
innermost being to the control of a Father God and a male priesthood. In the

schools of society's educational system, she is taught to glorify war and to accept the use of force and violence by men to dominate women and other men. She learns about gender roles—that women are to think, speak, behave, and carry themselves differently than men as she aspires to her maternal nurturing role. In the media, she sees herself mirrored in the serving roles that make the patriarchal culture work. In the polity, she is to be grateful that decisions are made by men because women can't think clearly enough about public issues. They may vote, preferably according to the views of the men of their family, but should be kept out of all but minor public offices. In the market place, she is to buy whatever the media have convinced her is neces-sary for her comfort and well-being. In the workplace, she is confined to the lowest-paying positions with the least opportunity for advancement—she is, after all, only supposed to work for pocket money for the household. Every space that women enter is dominated by male agents of the patriarchal order, telling them what to do and how to do it.

But there is another way to see the situation of woman. Figure 2 depicts her as a vibrant, active being at the center of a supportive circle of women's culture, a culture coextensive both with history and with the geographic space of the planet. For every one of the institutional spaces she inhabits, there is a set of women's networks to empower her, from planet-spanning international nongovernmental organizations with United Nations backing to local neigh-borhood support groups. They provide her with knowledge, skills, new ideas, political, economic, social, and spiritual support. In addition, most of all these networks affirm her as a person, a coshaper of the world she inhabits.

Now each institutional space becomes a medium for change. In the house-hold, women forge new egalitarian relationships with men, teaching their partners household and parenting skills, and preparing the next generation for a world in which gender does not define social roles. In the community of faith, the feminine aspect of the Godhead becomes visible. Women priests begin to provide a spiritual nurture that brings women and men to a new kind of spiritual maturity far beyond religious conformity. In schools, women as peace educators introduce the history of peacemaking and the skills of con-flict resolution in settings where all learning and action opportunities are equally open to boys and girls. The media also mirror an equal-opportunity world where women and minorities pioneer in new developments in the sciences and humanities, create social inventions which alter the character of social services and the patterns of organizational decisionmaking. Wherever women look, they can see themselves as doers. In the polity, they are sitting in increasing numbers in state legislatures and in courts; they control violence and fight fires and serve in society's regulatory and human services systems. They are courted as voters and their views are their own. In the market place,

Figure 2
The Agents of Social Transformation to the
Post-Patriarchal Order*

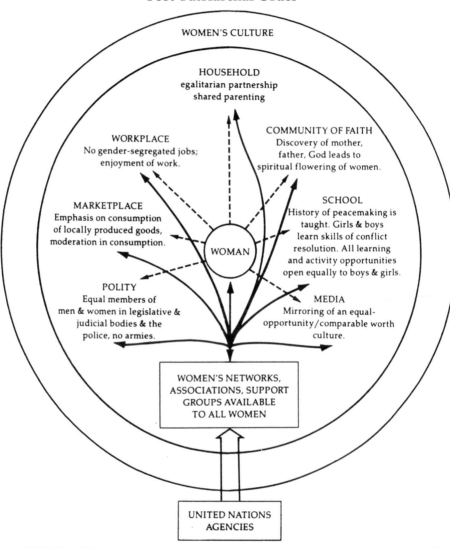

WOMEN'S CULTURE

HOUSEHOLD
egalitarian partnership
shared parenting

WORKPLACE
No gender-segregated jobs;
enjoyment of work.

COMMUNITY OF FAITH
Discovery of mother,
father, God leads to
spiritual flowering of women.

MARKETPLACE
Emphasis on consumption
of locally produced goods,
moderation in consumption.

SCHOOL
History of peacemaking is
taught. Girls & boys
learn skills of conflict
resolution. All learning
and activity opportunities
open equally to boys & girls.

WOMAN

POLITY
Equal members of
men & women in legislative &
judicial bodies & the
police, no armies.

MEDIA
Mirroring of an equal-
opportunity/comparable worth
culture.

WOMEN'S NETWORKS,
ASSOCIATIONS, SUPPORT
GROUPS AVAILABLE
TO ALL WOMEN

UNITED NATIONS
AGENCIES

* From E. Boulding, in Sakamoto, 1988.

they are insisting on new standards for consumer goods and food products and are creating new consumer protection devices. In the workplace, they are breaking out of gender-segregated jobs and providing leadership in every economic sector from commerce to the professions to the arts.

Which picture is true? Both. The patriarchal order does constrain women even while the women's culture empowers them. At this historical moment, however, I suggest that the old balance between the patriarchal culture and the women's culture is changing, and that something new is gradually emerging which promises a more humane, just, and peaceable future for both women and men.

THE 200-YEAR PRESENT

In order to understand the social changes of concern, we must consider a time span longer than the recent decades usually identified as a baseline for social development. The 200-year present begins June 17, 1888, the day of birth of those centenarians who are celebrating their hundredth birthday today. The other boundary of the 200-year present is June 17, 2088, when the babies born today will celebrate their hundredth birthday. This time span is directly accessible to us through the fact that our lives are intertwined with those of older folks we have known who were born in the 1880s, and our lives will be intertwined with those of children as yet unborn who will be alive in the 2080s. This period is neither ancient history nor distant future, it is our historical present. What is happening in this period is in a profound sense happening *to us.*

It helps us understand the 1980s if we know that the 1880s saw the beginning of the new era of global networks which have enabled women as well as men to act across national boundaries together with people of other continents on behalf of world rather than mere national interest. This was the great era of the new women's missionary movement enabling women to discover their world sisterhood, and the period in which the first transnational women's associations emphasizing peace, such as the Young Women's Christian Association and the Women's Christian Temperance Union, were formed. It was also the era in which the International Council of Nurses was formed. Nursing was the first profession to establish an international sisterhood specifically based on a professional calling.

The beginning of our 200-year present was an exciting time. It was the era of the grand European socialist-pacifist-feminist vision of a world without war, poverty, or injustice, which also spilled over into the Americas. There was Clara Zetkin in Germany, Rosa Luxembourg in Poland, Luisa Kautsky in Austria,

Vera Zasulich in Russia, Angelica Balabonov in Italy, and later Beatrice Webb in England, and Jane Addams in the United States. Because there was a lapse in the Grand Vision after two world wars and the depression of the 1930s, few of us today know how much we owe to those foremothers.

But the Grand Vision was not only found in Europe. In India, Kristo and Kumadini Mitter, Swami Kumari, Sarla Devi, and others led a movement to educate women to build a new India freed from colonial structures; China's "first woman revolutionary," Ch'iu Chin, joined Sun Yat Sen's political party and led the women's movement to free women from the bonds of ignorance; in Japan, there were the same stirrings, the same movement to liberate women from tradition; in Africa, tribal women were confronting colonial occupiers who were destroying the livelihood of their people. In Latin America, Maria Alvarado of Peru and Amanda Labarca of Chile were the more visible figures among the many Latin American professional women who were also political activists seeking a better situation for women in a more just society. It was these women from all continents who formed the first transnational women's networks for peace and justice, later formalized as international nongovernmental organizations. A special part of those networks consisted of women trained in law and the social sciences who developed the first peace education materials in the West and helped lay the foundations for the International Arbitration movement which led to the International Court of Justice, the League of Nations, and more recently the United Nations.

LAPSE AND RECOVERY OF VISION

Women had little energy for visioning in the war-depression-war decades from 1914 to 1945. Serving as nurses on battlefields, and eventually as soldiers in the ranks; working long hours at demanding factory jobs; feeding a family during long stretches of unemployment—these were not activities conducive to visioning. Betty Friedan's *Feminine Mystique* documents one aspect of those years, the retreat into the home. Women's organizations lost membership and sought simply to survive. But by the late 1960s women were coming to life again. They did not know what their grandmothers and greatgrandmothers had done, but they knew what they needed to do: replace a militaristic social order with an order that was nurturant of all living things, and do it by finding a place for women in the public sphere where opinions are formed and decisions made.

Now we are at midpoint in the 200-year present. Will this recovery of vision and activism last, or do we risk another women's retreat as happened in the second quarter of this century? There is reason to believe that women's new visibility in the public sphere will endure. The grand vision of the 1880s was shared by a small educated international sisterhood. Today increasing numbers of women on all continents have access to the tools needed for participation in the modern world. Here are some factors that give durability to the current opening up of opportunities for women as shapers of their world.

1. Education. Levels of literacy for women are steadily increasing. While for two-thirds of the world's women only elementary level education is available, the number of women entering secondary and university education is everywhere increasing. Sixty percent of the world's women were still illiterate in 1960; now only a little over one-third are illiterate, and the number continues to shrink. When women have access to knowledge of larger world, they will no longer suffer their controlled by those who do.

2. Labor force participation. While women have always been at least half of the world's labor force, today they are increasingly part of that part of the labor force which is counted and recognized. The number of women who are unpaid home workers is dwindling. This means more public regulation of working conditions for women as well as men. While generally women still earn only one-half of what men do, the trend is toward a narrowing of the gap, however slow.

3. Women elected officials. There is a worldwide trend of increased numbers of women elected to local and state/provincial governing councils, and a slower trend of election to national parliaments. This means that women are gaining experience in managing public affairs at the local level which will make them increasingly effective as they serve in national parliaments. At present some women who serve in national parliaments are elites without grassroots experience. This will change, however.

4. Women professionals. More women with university training means more women entering the professions in every country, and more women available for high-level public and private sector roles as planners and decisionmakers. This is most noticeable at the local level, where a coalition of women office holders and women professionals have been able to improve the quality of

health, education, and welfare services in many communities. The formation of similar coalitions at the national level will take longer, but it is happening. For the nursing profession, which has suffered as much as any profession from gender gaps in status and authority which prevent nurses from exercising their competence to improve health care, this kind of coalition building is very important.

5. The UN women's decade. The growth of international women's networks is part of a worldwide growth of people's networks which is already transforming the international system. In 1900, there were 50 states, many colonized areas, and several hundred international nongovernmental organizations. Today there are over 160 states, fewer colonies, and 18,000 nongovernmental organizations crisscrossing the old boundaries of nation states-cum-colonies.

The United Nations has played a special role in helping women and former colonies to find their places as full participants in the new international order. Looking back at Figure 2, you will see I have placed the UN in the diagram to show a relationship between the presence of the UN and the formation of women's networks internationally. The United Nations Women's Decade had the effect of making national governments allocate resources to bring women together to assess their situation. This has made possible the gradual development of an understanding and a degree of partnership between women of the South and North that did not exist before 1975. The Women's Decade gatherings were convened to assess very specific local realities in relation to equality, development, and peace. The three successive conferences in Mexico City (1975), in Copenhagen (1980), and in Nairobi (1985) brought women together in concrete working relationships with the opportunity to build on what had gone before and to plan for the future. There were 6,000 women present in Mexico City and 14,000 at the Nairobi conference ten years later.

During that same period, the women who participated in the Women's Decade activities formed 30 entirely new intercontinental women's networks directed to specific problems relating to equality, development, and peace. Table 1, which lists the names, founding event, and coordinating office of each network, gives some idea of the scope and character of these new organizations. In addition, there are several hundred women's international nongovernmental organizations that already existed in the 1970s. This is an impressive international mobilization of women's capabilities. What will be the result in the next half of our 200-year present?

Table 1
Some International Women's Networks Founded Since 1974*

1. 1974—IFN (International Feminist Network) [=, HR]
   Founding Event: International Tribunal on Crimes Against Women held in Brussels, Belgium in March, 1974 spawned the idea for IFN.
   Location: as of 1987, Rome, Italy.

2. 1974—ISIS International [=, D]
   Founding Event: ISIS International grew out of the perceived needs of women at the International Tribunal on Crimes Against Women.
   Location: as of 1987, Santiago, Chile and Rome, Italy.

3. 1975—IWTC (International Women's Tribune Centre) [=, D]
   Founding Event: Following the International Women's Year Nongovernmental Tribune held in Mexico City, 1975.
   Location: as of 1987, New York, New York, USA.

4. 1976—AAWORD (Association of African Women for Research and Development) [R, D]
   Founding Event: Lusaka, Zambia, Consultative Meeting of the Swedish Agency for Research Cooperation with Developing Countries in 1976.
   Location: In the country where the President resides.

5. 1979—GASAT (Girls and Science and Technology) [D]
   Founding Event: In 1979, informal meeting of concerned researchers to discuss their work in assisting access of girls and women to careers in scientific and technological fields. An international forum was proposed. Four subsequent international forums: Netherlands, 1981; Oslo, 1983; London, 1985; and Michigan, USA, 1987.
   Location: as of 1987, Ann Arbor, Michigan, USA.

6. 1979—WWB (Women's World Banking) [D]
   Founding Event: In 1979, under Netherlands law a not-for-profit Netherlands foundation was formed to promote women entrepreneurs around the world.
   Location: as of 1987, New York, New York, USA.

7. 1979—Women, Militarism, and Disarmament Study Group of the International Peace Research Association [P]
   Founding Event: Special meeting at the 1979 IPRA Conference for women members to discuss their research priorities and the problem of sexism in the conduct of peace research.
   Location: as of 1987, Santiago, Chile.

8. 1980—International Interdisciplinary Congress on Women [R]
   Founding Event: The first IIC on women was held in Israel in 1981.
   Location: as of 1986, Dublin, Ireland.

9. 1982—AWID (Association for Women in Development) [D]
   Founding Event: Created by a group of scholars, practitioners and policy makers in 1982. It is a US association linking to other national and regional associations outside the US.
   Location: as of 1987, Manhattan, Kansas, USA.

10. 1982—CAW (Committee for Asian Women) [=, D]
    Founding Event: Recognition of the need to support the struggle of Asian women workers began in 1977 in Malaysia at the Christian Conference of Asia-Urban Rural Mission. Through the work of many women in Tokyo, Taiwan, Bangladesh, India, Sri Lanka, Thailand, and Korea the idea of CAW kept building until it was affirmed in the Electronics Workshop in Malaysia in October 1981 and an organizing committee was held in Bangkok, Thailand, December, 1982.
    Location: as of 1985, Kowloon, Hong Kong.

11. 1983—WLD (Women, Law, and Development Program) [=, D]
Founding Event: OEF International committed itself in 1983 to a long-term program which would support through collaboration the number of women's groups working towards women's rights.
Location: as of 1987, Washington, DC, USA.

12. 1983—Sisterhood is Global Institute [=, D]
Founding Event: Project of compiling reports and data for *Sisterhood is Global,* lasting from late 1970s to 1983.
Location: as of 1987, New York, New York, USA.

13. 1984—International Feminist Book Fair [D, M]
Founding Event: in London in 1984.
Location: Tentatively planned for New Delhi, India, February 1988.

14. 1984—ISIS WICS (International Women's Information and Communication Service) [D, M]
Founding Event: Isis International created two branches in 1984: ISIS-WICS, Women's Information and Communication Service and ISIS-WICCE, Women's International Cross-Cultural Exchange.
Location: as of 1987, Rome, Italy, and Santiago, Chile.

15. 1984—Latin American and Caribbean Women and Health Network [D, H]
Founding Event: The first Regional Women and Health Meeting organized by the Corporacion Regional para el desarroilo integral de la Mujer y law Familia (Bogota, Colombia) was held in May 1984.
Location: as of 1987, Santiago, Chile.

16. 1984—Women Living Under Muslim Laws [=, HR]
Founding Event: An informal meeting of Muslim women in Europe in 1984 met to discuss the misinterpretation of Islam by men and the state which suppress women's basic human rights. First formal organized meeting was in Aragon, France, in April, 1986.
Location: as of 1987, Combaillaux, France.

17. 1986—CAFRA (Caribbean Association for Feminist Research and Action) [R, D]
Founding Event: In 1980, in Puerto Rico women activists and scholars from around the Caribbean attended IDS/CEREP (Institute of Development Studies, University of Sussex-Centro de Estudios de la Realidad Puertoriquena) seminar on women and social production in the Caribbean.
Location: as of 1987, St. Augustine, Trinidad and Tobago.

18. 1985—DAWN (Development Alternatives with Women for a New Era) [R, D]
Founding Event: 1985 UN World Women's Conference in Nairobi at the NGO's Forum: women researchers, activists, and policy makers presented a position paper outlining the creation of DAWN.
Location: as of July, 1987, Botafago, Brazil, region changes every two years.

19. 1985—GROOTS (Grass Roots Organizations Operating Together For Sisterhood) [D]
Founding Event: Network begun in Nairobi among low-income rural women and women workers.
Location: as of 1987, Mylapore, Madras, India.

20. 1985—IWDA (International Women's Development Agency) [D]
Founding Event: Agency grew in part from the Australian Women and Development Network.
Location: as of 1987, Victoria, Australia.

21. 1985—World Women Parliamentarians for Peace [P]
Founding Event: Meeting to support initiatives of superpowers toward disarmament in 1985.
Location: as of 1987, New Delhi, India.

22. 1985—Women for a Meaningful Summit, International Liaison Office [P]
    Founding Event: Began as ad hoc coalition of women and organizations active in arms control in the US in August, 1985.
    Location: as of 1987, Athens, Greece.

23. 1986—Third World Movement Against the Exploitation of Women [=, HR]
    Founding Event: April 1986 gathering of peace, disarmament, women's, and church groups resulted in a new campaign: the Campaign Against Military Prostitution, CAMP International.
    Location: as of 1987, contact in Manila, Philippines.

24. 1986—Arab Women Solidarity Association [=, HR]
    Founding Event: Created in early 1986.
    Location: as of 1987, Cairo, Egypt.

25. 1986—Asian Pacific Women Action Network
    Founding Event: Resulted from a training program in Bangkok in April, 1986, sponsored by the Asian Cultural Forum on Development.
    Location: as of 1987, Bangkok, Thailand.

26. 1986—WINGS (Women's International News Gathering Service) [D, M]
    Founding Event: Sponsored by Western Public Radio, a nonprofit audio production and training facility.
    Location: as of 1987, San Francisco, California, USA.

27. 1986—Women, Environment and Sustainable Development Network [D, ENV]
    Founding Event: Nairobi NGO Forum spawned a series of preparatory activities of women's organizations and environmental groups resulting in the 1986 Network.
    Location: as of 1987, Amsterdam, Netherlands.

28. 1986—Womenwealth [=, D]
    Founding Event: After Nairobi, in response to the many calls for North-South cooperation among women.
    Location: as of 1987, London, England.

29. 1987—Feminist Futures International Network
    Founding Event: Symposium at Siuntio Baths, Finland on "Women and the Military System."
    Location: Temporary (first two issues, 1987) Boulder, Colorado, USA.

30. 1987—Global Fund For Women [D]
    Founding Event: The Board of Directors of the Global Fund For Women met in Spring 1987 in response to the Nairobi Conference call to governments, NGOs, and individuals to take specific steps to improve the status of women.
    Location: To be determined.

Category Code Key:

D	Development	D, M	Development, Media
=, D	Equality and Development	D, H	Development, Health
=, HR	Equality and Human Rights	D, ENV	Development, Environment
R, D	Research, Development	P	Peace

Code is indicated in [ ] at the end of each Network Title.

* From E. Boulding in Sakamote, 1988.

THE NEW VISION

The new international women's movement has taken the ingredients of the Grand Vision of a century ago and translated it into a process model. Yet what must be in place for there to be peace, justice, and a humane way of living in the 21st century for all people, including women? Here is a highly abbreviated summary of what the new feminists have to say about peace, equality, and development, three themes important in the Grand Vision of the 1880s and also central to the UN Women's Decade vision.

Peace

In the old Grand Vision, disarmament and stopping wars were a primary focus. In the new approach, focus has shifted to the phenomenon of domination and its undergirding patriarchal institutions. The new feminist message specifies that there cannot be peace in the world as long as there is violence against women. This linkage of micro and macro processes is one of the major insights contemporary feminism has added to older feminist thinking about the abolition of war.

Equality

Along with ending war, equality was a key theme in the old Grand Vision. Yet getting the vote and associated legal and property rights did little for women's status in the workforce and little to move women into policymaking positions. The new feminism has produced a veritable army of women lawyers around the world who work on the specifics of human rights for women as detailed in the 21 UN conventions on the rights of women, country by country. The new feminism has also propelled women into political office in a way undreamed of 100 years ago, which moves them closer to public decisionmaking, although the road ahead is still long and fraught with difficulty.

Development

The Grand Vision of the 1880s was concerned with urban and rural poverty and social misery, particularly as it struck women. The concept of social and economic development as a multifaceted phenomenon involving every aspect of society and every level of activity from the home to the international marketplace, however, was not conceived of by women or men at that time. Mainstream male postwar thinking about economic development for newly independent and less industrialized countries has on the whole been arid and led to a widening of the poverty gap between North and South. The new feminism has shown the emptiness of development plans based on "take-off" or "trickle-down" theories of investing primarily in a country's industrial base, including the industrialization of agriculture.

Through painful struggles during the Women's Decade, the international sisterhood has forged an understanding of development as *human* development, taking account of great cultural differences and highly varied economic and political situations from region to region around the world. Feminism has also shown the centrality of woman to development, as farmer and food provider, healer, child bearer, teacher, water and wood carrier, home builder, weaver, pottery and artifact producer, and organizer of markets. Policymakers are still slow to include women's expertise in planning, but a new awareness is beginning. Most of the 30 new women's networks listed in Table 1 deal with some aspect of development, and with the issue of putting women's expertise to work in humanizing development.

Ecofeminism

The old Grand Vision did not include much about the environment—the warning signals of serious environmental deterioration were yet to appear. (It should be noted however that the term *ecology* was indeed first used by a woman, Ellen Swallow, in 1892.) The new feminism sees the destruction of the natural environment as an aspect of the patriarchal order. Ecofeminism is a manifestation of postpatriarchal consciousness, politically embodied in the Green movement. It is no accident that women provide the major leadership for the Greens in the 10 or so countries that have Green political parties.

Ecofeminism is equally strong in the countries of the North and the South. It espouses decentralization, nonviolence, community participation in shaping the conditions of life locally, small-scale enterprises, and the use of appropriate and resource-conserving technologies in agriculture and industry. Ecofeminism also provides a home for the feminist movement toward holistic healing. It has a strong spiritual component, and a heightened awareness of the feminine aspects of the Creator. The lesbian way of life, witnessing in a special way to the wholeness of women, also finds an acceptance in ecofeminism that it does not always find elsewhere in the women's movement.

Ecofeminism is both the most inclusive and the most extreme statement of the new vision. Most feminists will accept some part of the ecofeminist vision, but few will accept it in its entirety. Nevertheless, it is important as a statement of new directions for the next century.

THE GROUNDS FOR HOPE

Each of the elements contributed by the new feminism to the building of a new social order listed above has some grounding in the old Grand Vision. We owe a lot to our foremothers. But we must also acknowledge how much ground was lost in mid-century. I am suggesting that the reasons for hope at this midpoint in the 200-year present is that the new women's movement brings so much to the work of world-shaping that was not available to our foremothers. Currently working from a more solid base, our gains may not be so easily lost.

There is also a new sophistication in world view. First, women see interconnections between aspects of social and economic life both within and between societies that we did not understand before. There are the skills of networking, and the infrastructures of women's organizations to work with, as well as interconnections with the rest of the 18,000 international nongovernmental organizations that help shape the modern world.

Second, the level of professional and political know-how of women makes new levels of inventiveness possible. Every aspect of the old social order needs reworking, from education, healing, and human welfare to eco. omic and governance structures. In each of these arenas women bring new ways of working, substantively new approaches to nurturing human potentiality, and skill in developing organizational forms that are not the victim of bureaucratic complexity. The inventiveness of women in the healing professions, particularly in nursing, far outstrip society's capacity to absorb that inventiveness. While this is discouraging for nursing, it calls for the making of alliances with women politicians and planners to overcome the resistance of male traditionalists. This is already beginning to happen in Colorado, and I celebrate the new alliances!

Third, women now have a healthy self-awareness of nurturant styles of performing in their professional and public roles which are at the same time autonomous and self-respecting, as distinct from earlier styles of subservient nurturance which the women's movement has properly rejected. This is still a subject of keen debate—how "maternalist" should women be? How develop nurturant rules which do not, however, nurture patriarchy? There are still rewards for "playing the game" and succeeding as "female men," but the balance of thinking points to taking responsibility for the creation of new models of nurturance, new standards for mutuality of social relationships, in both public and private social roles.

Fourth, women are rediscovering children after a long period of absorption in their own development needs. Now that child care is a central issue for women, the development of children can receive the same attention that the development of women has been receiving. These are, of course, two sides of the same coin. The new focus on children offers the opportunity to open up for boys as well as girls, from an early age, a fuller range of their own potentials. It is they who will be living out the new social roles we are now inventing.

While I am emphasizing grounds for hope that women will be more fully involved in shaping the new social order of the 21st century, that involvement will not be automatic. Knowing what we have to work with, assessing the developing our own capabilities, having confidence in our own inventiveness, and all preconditions for bringing to reality in the second half of the 200-year present the ecofeminist vision described earlier. But the most important condition of all is being willing to work for the vision in our own daily lives. Action without vision can be trivial, but vision without action is a betrayal of human possibility.

REFERENCES

Boulding, E., Nuss, S., Carson, D., & Greenstein, M. (1976) *Handbook of international data on women.* New York, Sage Publications, Halsted Press/John Wiley.

Caldecott, L., & Leland, S. (eds.) (1983) *Reclaim the earth.* London: The Women's Press.

Flammang, J. (1984) *Political women, current roles in state and local government.* Beverly Hills: Sage Yearbooks in Women's Policy Studies.

International Centre for Parliamentary Documentation. (1988) *Participation of women in political life and in the decision-making process.* Geneva: Inter-Parliamentary Union.

International Women's Tribune Center. (1983) *Rights of women. A workbook of international conventions relating to women's issues and concerns.* New York: International Women's Tribune Center.

Schuler, M. *Empowerment and the law, strategies of third world women.* Washington DC: OEF International.

Seager, J., & Olson, A. *Women in the world: An international atlas.* New York: Simon & Schuster.

United Nations. (1980) *World conference to review and appraise the achievements of the United Nations decade for women: Equality, development and peace,* Nairobi, Kenya, 15-26 July, 1985. A. Conference 116/28. New York: United Nations.

United Nations. (1987) *World statistics in brief. United Nations satistical pocketbook.* (11th ed.) Department of International Economic and Social Affairs, Statistical Office, Statistical Papers Series V, No. 11. New York: United Nations.

3

Looking at Caring and Nursing Through a Feminist Lens

Kathleen I. MacPherson

I believe nursing cannot become self-directing or effective in the politics of care without embracing feminism and all it stands for.

Jo Ann Ashley, 1980.

The two concepts of caring and nursing occupy a central place in the way nurses attempt to describe what is unique about our profession. The linking of caring to nursing has become an ideology that stresses the uniqueness and essentiality of our work. We have also obviously reached the public with this message. In the May 23, 1988 issue of *Newsweek*, George F. Will wrote in his column titled "The Dignity of Nursing" that "the American ideal of a doctor— kindly, caring, reassuring Dr. Welby—was essentially a nurse" (p. 80).

On the other hand, Sara T. Fry has written a compelling article, "The Ethic of Caring: Can it Survive in Nursing?", in *Nursing Outlook*, January 1987. As we are recognizing, along with the public, that caring is a central ethic of nursing, we are also recognizing that our ability to operationalize this ethic is being seriously undermined by the social context in which we practice.

Within nursing, caring has developed into an ethic as a result of several influences. An historical influence is Nightingale's definition of nursing practice found in *Notes on Nursing* (1859) as: "[being] in charge of somebody's health . . . to put the patient in the best condition for nature to act upon him [sic]." Hildegard Peplau's 1952 ground-breaking book, *Interpersonal Relations in Nursing: A Conceptual Frame of Reference for Psychodynamic Nursing,* taught nurses to care by the therapeutic use of self. Madeleine M. Leininger, Jean Watson, and other nurse scholars have also had a more contemporary influence on the development of the caring ethic in nursing.

THE CARING ETHIC IN NURSING

Madeleine M. Leininger began the first cross-cultural study of care in the early 1960s. In her book, *Transcultural Nursing: Concepts, Theories and Practices* (1978), she defined caring in terms of nurturant and skillful activities, processes, and decisions to assist people on their own terms. Her other book, *Care: The Essence of Nursing and Health* (1984), addresses philosophic, theoretical, research, and applied aspects of caring.

Jean Watson in her two books, *Nursing: The Philosophy and Science of Caring* (1979) and *Nursing: Human Science and Human Care: A Theory of Nursing* (1985), views caring as a humanistic and interpersonal process that is essential for a therapeutic relationship between the nurse and client. Watson makes a clear distinction between medicine's curing the patient of disease and nursing's caring processes that help the patient attain or maintain health, or die a peaceful death. She has articulated some basic premises for the science of caring in nursing and 10 primary carative factors that form the structure for studying and understanding nursing as the science of caring. Watson views the act of transpersonal caring in nursing as a human art, a human science, and a moral ideal (1985, p. 68).

Other nurse scholars have participated in the development of a science of caring by presenting papers at the National Research Caring Conferences and the National Transcultural Nursing Care Conferences, by publishing, and by conducting research. For example, Delores Gaut has contributed a philosophic orientation to caring research, a theoretical description of caring as action, and a method for evaluating caring competencies in nursing practice. Marilyn Ray has applied caring theory to nursing practice in her paper "The Development of a Classification System of Institutional Caring" (1984).

It appears that a new trend emerged at the Tenth National Research Care Conference held May 1-3, 1988. Deborah S. Bockman presented a paper "Nurturing the Human Spirit in the Work Place: Caring for the Nurse" and Mary Lou Sheston spoke on "Caring in Nursing Education: The Development of a Construct." We are beginning to acknowledge our own need for caring, and our students' need for caring before we can care for others.

The present paradigm of caring and nursing is based on a scientific and humanistic foundation—no doubt, we have come a long way. Today I suggest, however, that we infuse a strong element of feminist theory to the philosophical, scientific, and transcultural perspectives that underpin our current caring and nursing paradigm.

Susan Reverby, in *Ordered to Care* (1987), has written that the central dilemma of American nursing is the order to care in a society that refuses to value caring. To explore the meaning of caring for nursing, it is necessary to unravel the relationship between nursing and womanhood which has been formed over the last century. Reverby's work as well as that of Barbara Melosh (1982), author of *The Physician's Hand*, and JoAnn Ashley (1976), author of *Hospitals, Paternalism and the Role of the Nurse*, can greatly enhance our understanding of nursing history from a feminist perspective. As a result, we will explore how to build on the theoretical work that has been done on caring and nursing by way of feminist theory.

FEMINIST THEORY AS A LENS

Feminist theory focuses on aspects of caring largely missing in the existing paradigm. The current paradigm stresses individual motivation for caring while ignoring both the material conditions and power relations in the contexts where nurses work.

Usually defined as an active desire to change women's position in society, feminism also encompasses the view that it is a social movement for change in the position of women. At the very least, a feminist is someone who believes that women suffer discrimination because of their sex. The philosopher Sandra Lee Bartky (1977) states:

> To be a feminist, one first has to become one often through a profound personal transformation. The feminist changes behavior and changes consciousness. She sees a new "social reality" as the scales fall from her eyes. She sees how women are oppressed in the family, in the workplace and in society. Through this understanding, it is possible for her to work with other women for liberation. (pp. 22–23)

Because feminist claims touch every aspect of our lives, the term *feminism* carries a potential emotional ch. rge. For some it is merely pejorative; for others it is an honor to be known as a feminist.

Contemporary feminism has many faces. Therefore, when we use a feminist lens, we will see variations in feminist theories of oppression and in the solutions proposed for eliminating such oppression. These theories are usually played off against the traditional or conservative theoretical view of women's situation in society, which denies that women are oppressed. In addition, the conservative view defends women's position as it is by arguing for its supposed natural, even biological and social imperative. Psychoanalytic and sociobiological theories are often used to support the position.

According to radical feminists, this conservative view of women's situation arises from a patriarchal order which exists in all societies regardless of political persuasion. Patriarchy is a "socially constructed reality" that values men more than women and which gives men more status and prestige simply because they are men (Gray, 1982). Men have institutionalized advantages over women in almost every sphere.

Alison Jagger (1983), a feminist political philosopher, offers feminist theories as "ideal types" that minimize the similarities between them and sharpen the differences. When such theories are compared with each other, the understanding of each is deepened and a sense of the ongoing and dialectical process of feminist theorizing emerges.

Feminist theories define the causes of women's oppression and offer a means for eliminating it. Historically, the theories have developed in the following order: liberal, radical, and socialist feminist.

Liberal Feminism

Liberal feminism is the most widely diffused and generally acceptable version of feminism. It stresses equality of opportunity for women. Social inequalities in wealth, position, and power are not criticized as such, but liberal feminists believe that women should be able to compete with men on an equal basis. The roots of women's oppression are seen to lie in a lack of equal civil rights and educational opportunities. There is no attempt at historical analysis to discover why such a lack should exist. Instead, it is believed that women's oppression can be dealt with by attacking sexist discrimination. This theory equates the elimination of sexist discrimination with women's liberation.

Betty Friedan's *The Feminine Mystique* expressed the liberal feminist position which was then given organizational form in the National Organization for Women (NOW). In creating the present caring and nursing paradigm that emphasizes an ethic of caring from a primarily individualistic orientation, the work of a few liberal feminists was selectively used. Gilligan (1982) and Noddings (1984) exemplify this view of caring.

Essentially, Gilligan's work is a revisionist attempt to prove that Kolberg's concept of stages of human moral development (which placed men at a level higher than women) was flawed, based as it was on a totally male research sample. Gilligan claims that women tend to define themselves in terms of the context of their relationships. They are drawn to the role of caretaker and nurturer, often putting their own needs at the bottom of the list, preceded by other people: husband, children, or their own parents. This leads to a moral imperative to care, to be responsible for discerning and alleviating the real and recognizable trouble of this world. For men, the moral imperative appears as an injunction to respect the rights of others and to protect from interference their own rights to life and self-fulfillment. For Gilligan, however, through caring women connect emotionally with others while through dependence on laws and rights men isolate themselves emotionally.

Nel Noddings (1984) argues that human caring and the memory of caring and being cared for form the foundation of ethical response itself. Caring here is a reciprocal process between the "one-caring" and the "cared-for":

> *Caring involves stepping out of one's own personal frame of reference into the other's. When we care, we consider the other's point of view, his objective needs, and what he expects of us. Our attention, our mental engrossment is on the cared for, not on ourselves. Our reasons for acting, then, have to do both with the other's wants and desires and with the objective elements of his problematic situation.* (p. 24)

As liberal feminists, Gilligan and Noddings have acknowledged caring as the highest level of moral development.

Caring characterizes nurses' work and is seen by nurses as inappropriately undervalued in the larger society. It is little wonder that nursing leaders found Gilligan's and Noddings' work acceptable for incorporation into their paradigm of caring and nursing. One must speculate, however, on how engrossment (as discussed by Noddings) and an I–them relationship as discussed by Watson can be applied to nurses' relationship with clients in our current social context (Mishler, 1979).

A second form of liberal feminist activism of importance for nurses was the surge in literature critical of medicine's treatment of women patients. Nurses exposed to this literature became aware of "blind spots" in their professional education. For example, wife battering had not been connected to depression or suicide. Literature of cesarean sections (Arms, 1975) diethystilbesterol (DES) (Seaman and Seaman, 1977), breast cancer (Kushner, 1975), hysterectomies (Morgan, 1982), menopause (Voda, Dinnerstein, & O'Donnell, 1982; MacPherson, 1981) osteoporosis (MacPherson, 1985), and mental illness (Chesler, 1972) gave nurses familiar with this literature the opportunity to care for their women patients by explaining the risks inherent in certain medical, surgical, and psychiatric treatments.

Third, liberal feminists have used the courts to fight for abortion rights, and for retribution for women damaged by medical treatments such as DES and the Dalcon Shield. They have fought to get more women in law and medicine to humanize these professions. Some feminists also desire an increase in the population of men in nursing as a means of addressing the problem of a sex-segregated profession.

Liberal feminism appears to provide nursing with a political language that argues for equality and rights within the given order of things. It suggests a basis for caring that stresses individual discretion and values, acknowledging that the nurse's right to care should be given equal consideration with the physician's right to cure. Reverby (1987) states:

> *Classical liberalism's tenets applied to women have much to offer nursing. The demand for the right to care questions deeply held beliefs about gendered relations in the health care hierarchy and the structure of the hierarchy itself.* (p. 10)

However, liberal feminist theory is limited in its explanation of why many nurses find themselves forced to abandon the effort to care, or nursing altogether. From a feminist perspective, the individualism and autonomy promised by this rights framework often fails to acknowledge collective social need, to provide a way for adjudicating conflicts over rights, or to address the reasons for the devaluing of female activity. The following example illustrates such limitations.

Lemons et al. v. the City and County of Denver was a pay equity case brought by ten nurses against their employers in April 1978. These nurses argued that they were discriminated against in the city's job classification system (one of the first comparable worth cases). Judge Fred Winner heard the case without a jury and decided that the city was not in violation of Title VII of the Civil Rights Act of 1964. In effect, Judge Winner stated that history had created a lower wage scale for some occupations. Judge Winner also indicated that he felt constrained to rule against the nurses because a favorable ruling would have had the potential for "disrupting the entire economic system of the United States of America." The case was appealed in 1981 and the lower court's decision was upheld, although it was acknowledged that nurses had a legitimate concern but without recourse under the present system to correct it. The U.S. Supreme Court refused to hear an appeal to correct pay inequities. The ten nurses who were seeking a fair salary in order to care for their own needs were denied their equal rights by three levels of the judicial system.

Radical Feminism

Currently, while radical feminism is the least developed and systematic of all feminist theory, it is also the most original. It does not draw from previously existing social or economic theories; rather, it is being developed from a woman-centered worldview by women themselves (Chinn & Wheeler, 1985). The major theoretical and philosophical work to date defines itself by challenging the existing concepts and language of patriarchal systems and by formulating concepts derived from a woman-identified perspective (Daly, 1978).

Radical feminists assert that the oppression of women is fundamental to all types of economic systems—from capitalist to socialist—and cannot be removed by economic and social changes alone such as the abolition of class society. On a more personal level, qualitatively as well as quantitatively, women's oppression also causes the most suffering to its victims, although such suffering may go unrecognized due to the sexist prejudices of both oppressors and victims. As a result, women's liberation requires the abolition of institutionalized gender discrimination. For some theorists such as Firestone, this liberation extends to the extrauterine reproduction of children, a medical procedure whose systematic use must be considered a distinct possibility. Other radical theorists question cultural institutions believed to play a major role in women's oppression: the family, prostitution, and pornography.

The primary distinction of radical feminism, however, is its view of women's relationship to man (Chinn & Wheeler, 1985). Liberal and socialist feminists define women in relation to men, even when proposing a new system. For example, "equality" from a liberal feminist view means "equal to men," and from a socialist perspective, "equal to men without class distinctions."

Radical feminist goals are not to achieve equality with men under existing social and economic structures, but to entirely transform social institutions. The critical feature of radical feminism is its starting point—discovering, analyzing, and valuing women's experience without the imposed standards of male ideology or systems (Chinn & Wheeler, 1985).

Through a radical feminist lens the medical profession is seen as yet another system which conforms to the patriarchal pattern established by the modern family. As Fee (1982) aptly states, the doctor-father runs a family composed of the nurse (wife and mother) and the patient (the child). The doctor possesses the scientific and technical skills and the nurse performs all caring duties. In response, radical feminists work to increase women's knowledge of their bodies so that women can question physicians about tests (such as mammograms), have access to their medical records, get names and descriptions of drugs being given, and so forth.

Other radical feminists' innovations in health care include self-help women's health groups (self-pelvic exams) and feminist health centers which are owned and controlled by women. Radical feminists can help nurses and other health care workers become aware of the deficiencies in the health delivery system generally. Radical feminists also have been leaders in inventing new forms of women-controlled organizations such as rape crisis centers, battered women's shelters, and women's communes that are based on collective rather than bureaucratic structures (Ferguson, 1984).

Kathleen Barry, sociologist author of *Female Sexual Slavery* (1979), exemplifies a pertinent instance of radical feminist theory and praxis. Barry defines female sexual slavery as present in all situations where women or girls cannot change the immediate conditions of their existence; where, regardless of how they got into these conditions, they cannot get out; and where they are subject to sexual violence and exploitation. Battered women, incest victims, and prostitutes are among the victims of female sexual slavery that Barry speaks of.

To combat this particularly women's problem, in 1980 Barry founded the International Feminist Network Against Female Sexual Slavery. In 1983, the Network met in Rotterdam where women from 24 countries discussed specific instances of forced prostitution, traffic in women, torture of female prisoners, sex tourism, military brothels, sexual mutilation, and other crimes against women. Immediately they discovered that the commonality of the oppression of women globally had created the basis for international feminist action.

In the United States, Barry argues for women-controlled shelters that provide safety and support for battered women, for teenage incest victims, and for prostitutes who want to escape sexual slavery. Barry's work thus points the way for nurses to become more caring about women who are victims of sexual violence. For example, nurses in emergency rooms need to practice professional caring and autonomy by referring these women to women shelters and rape crisis centers. Nurses can help the battered woman, the teenage incest victim, or the prostitute "take the first step" by calling a representative from a women's organization to come to the emergency room to talk to her. Emergency room nurses can also cooperate with Battered Women's Shelters and Rape Crisis Centers to provide training for other hospital nurses to recognize various forms of abuse against women and to be aware of community resources.

Connors (1980) and Lovell (1980) offer other examples of radical feminist analysis being applied to caring and nursing. Both address medical dominance, the silencing of nursing, medicine as iatrogenic, and the abusive care of women by physicians. Drawing on the work of Daly (1978), author of *Gyn/Ecology: The Metaethics of Radical Feminism*, Connors discusses the role of the nurse as token torturer. The role is expressed in part by "the nurse witnessing and/or participating in unnecessary and/or harmful treatments or surgery and by administering health-damaging drugs."

For women, the potential for suffering the iatrogenic affects of medical drugs is high. For example, DES given to prevent miscarriage caused vaginal cancer in some exposed mother's daughters and increased risk of breast cancer in the mothers themselves. The long-term effects of hormone replacement therapy, widely used to treat menopausal changes and prevent osteoporosis, are unknown. Nurses need to care enough about their women patients to reject the role of token torturer in silently and uncritically carrying out iatrogenic physicians' orders.

A third contribution that radical feminists can make to understand caring and nursing addresses nurses' relationships with each other. Does support, friendship, and caring exist among nurses, or do forms of "horizontal violence" with nurse pitted against nurse dominate our work settings? Chinn, Wheeler, Ray, and Wheeler published a questionnaire in the *American Journal of Nursing*, November 1987, designed to explore how friendships among nurses influence their personal and professional lives. The results support the theoretical framework found in Janice Raymond's *A Passion for Friends: Toward a Philosophy of Female Affection*. Findings indicate that obstructions to nurses' friendships were statistically significant.

At least one nurse scholar, Thompson (1987) has combined critical social theory with radical feminist theory to help nurses address sources of power and domination. She sees the need for critical scholars in nursing to present a systematic and thorough critique that uncovers hidden sources of "coercion, powerover, and domination" that are embedded in nurses' daily lived experience.

Despite such research, a radical feminist analysis of the existing paradigm of caring and nursing still remains to be done. The concept of ethical caring, built as it is on philosophical and transcultural nursing theory, does not incorporate the concepts of patriarchy and misogyny to help explicate common women's health problems such as depression, nor does it help to inform nurses of uncaring roles such as that of "token torturers."

Without a radical feminist analysis, nurses can be seduced into thinking that their relationship with physicians has become more equal when doctors decide that nurses need to "expand their role" or "collaborate more with physicians." It is only the liberal feminist who believes that with more courses and more degrees that doctors will treat nurses as equals.

Socialist Feminism

Socialist feminist theory accepts the historical materialist approach of Marx and Engels but seeks to enrich it by adding a class analysis of cultural institutions that play a major role in oppressing women: the family, motherhood, housework, and consumption.

Socialist feminists are committed to understanding the system of power deriving from capitalist patriarchy. As defined by Eisenstein (1979), capitalist patriarchy is characterized by the mutually reinforcing dialectical relationship between capitalist class structure and hierarchial sexual structuring. For example, patriarchal assumptions about women's role as wife and mother support and reinforce an economic system that pays women lower wages than men for the same work. In this view, capitalism cannot free itself from dependence on sexism any more than it can transcend class oppression or the pursuit of private profit. As a result, women will not be able freely to determine the condition of their own lives without eliminating the double oppression of a classist society and institutionalized gender discrimination.

Let us now look at the American health system through a socialist feminist lens. Here, the health system mirrors the organization of the larger system in its intense concentration of financial and political power on top, in its thoroughgoing stratification of its workforce by class, sex, and race, in its division of labor and specialization, in its very definitions of health and illness, and in its lack of accountability to the American people whom it theoretically serves (Fee, 1983).

Power is concentrated at the top of a hierarchy in a coalition that includes the American Medical Association and the commercial insurance companies. The great teaching hospitals and research institutions are dominated by representatives of the corporate class whereas the voluntary community hospitals are controlled by boards composed of upper-middle class professionals—doctors, lawyers, and business men predominate. Nurses, members of minority groups, and representatives of organized or unorganized labor are virtually excluded from access to any of these decision-making bodies.

Far below the capitalists are the lower-middle and working classes of the health industry. The former comprise most nurses and paraprofessional auxiliary and service personnel representing 54.2 percent of the total health labor force. (Fee, 1983). Both groups are predominantly female.

Greenleaf (1980), in an article titled "Sex-Segregated Occupations: Relevance for Nursing," spelled out the economics of sexual discrimination which form the basis for occupational segregation. In the sex-segregated health occupations these middle and working class groups are often played off against one another—nurse against nurse, licensed practical nurse (LPN), certified nurse assistant (CNA), and now registered care technologist (RCT). The RCT is a new category of health worker currently being socially constructed by the American Medical Association.

The non-physician workers are divided into over 375 independent occupations, most dead-end, low-wage positions. This process of continually bifurcating labor so as to parcel it out to a single worker is a general tendency of modern capitalism. Such fragmentation, as Braverman (1974) shows, is not to increase efficiency but to maximize management control over labor, and to replace highly skilled workers with less skilled and thus less costly workers.

If capitalist medicine fragments the organization of work, it also fragments the delivery of health care. It offers high-quality service to the wealthy, assembly-line care to the poor. Specialization makes it difficult, at almost any level, to find comprehensive care. In addition, social causes of illness such as asbestos dust in factories, or coal soot in mines, are largely ignored. Instead, the ideology of health promotion (which focuses on middle-class people) distracts the public's attention from the social causes of disease such as poverty, homelessness, unemployment, or underemployment.

Socialist feminist theory can be explored as a means of understanding several of the dilemmas in caring. Socialist feminists argue against an ahistorical interpretation of caring and instead present caring for others as historically created under particular circumstances, ideologies, and power relations (Graham, 1983). Caring is viewed as highly skilled emotional and physical work, in effect "a labor of love." With this description, Graham (1983), a British researcher on health policy, reminds us that all women are expected to do caring work. "As the providers of health, women are responsible for securing the domestic conditions necessary for the maintenance of health and for recovery from sickness" (p. 26).

In addition, Graham also addresses the politics of caring. She views the experience of women as health providers as contextually political. In particular, Graham examines recent developments in British health policy which shifts the burden of caring from the public to the private domain.

In the United States, the "nursing crisis" is an issue related essentially to caring. If nurses care, why are they leaving the profession? Reasons such as the women's movement's influence on women's access to other professions like medicine and law have been offered. A socialist feminist analysis would reject such an answer as insignificant and look instead to an analysis of the U.S. health system as a whole.

Throughout this century profit has been an underlying force for health sector development. During the past 15 years, health care has been increasingly corporatized by the medical-industrial complex which includes large investor-owned hospital chains such as Humana Corporation and Hospital Corporation of America, nursing homes, health maintenance organizations and ambulatory centers. (Salmon, 1987). Nurses and all other health care workers in these settings have been affected by the increasing emphasis on profit generation. Institutionalized control mechanisms such as diagnosis related groups (DRGs) and patient classification system (PCSs) with acronyms such as "GRASP" influence nurses' ability to care. Most recently, a plan by the American Medical Association to create RCTs is a further example of de-skilling nursing care. Recruitment is aimed at minorities that can be trained in a minimum of nine months to provide support for physicians' increasingly high technological interventions in hospitals.

As we know, hospital nurses are currently expected to "care" for more sicker patients than ever before, patients who are often discharged quicker. In such a social context, a socialist feminist would say that it is difficult, if not impossible, for nurses to operationalize an ethic of caring.

While some health care administrators may agree that working conditions for nurses should improve, wage and benefit packages increase, and so forth, the profit-oriented climate may make these options unrealistic (Moccia, 1987). Moccia suggests that these activities should be supported but that we need to see them as palliative measures.

In contrast to liberal feminists who are attempting to resolve the crisis in health care and the "nursing shortage" by improving the image and status of nurses, a group of socialist feminist nurses identifies the basic problem as the profit driven and sexist health care system. This group, Nurses for Progressive Social Change, believes that rather than problems with image and compensation, nurses' fundamental problems involve contradictions between their mission to care for people and a system that, while ostensibly for that purpose, obstructs nurses' opportunities to deliver nursing care (Moccia, 1987). If, as Moccia states, the crisis in the supply of nurses is related to the structure of the health care system and, through it, to larger social issues, we might best channel our efforts to resolve the nursing crisis by analyzing the relationships between the crisis in nursing, health care, and society. Socialist feminists also believe that nurses need to care for themselves and their patients through using collective bargaining for adequate wages and for obtaining a work context where caring is possible.

Federal cost-containment measures have targeted already limited resources for providing patient care for further reductions. Such measures will have a dramatic impact on personal interactions between nurses and their clients. Nurses will have less time to see the end results of nursing care plans or to make home visits. Nurses will have less and less control over the nature and scope of their work. As a result, it will become even more difficult to recruit and retain nurses and nursing students who are looking for opportunities to work with and care for people.

Adherents to the rich and complex feminist theories described continue to force lively debates in the women's movement as a whole. While nursing has not been in the forefront of activism in the women's movement of this century, nurses have benefited (1) from the liberal feminist view that uncovers realities of unequal opportunity and (2) from the socialist view that sustains many nurses' labor unions. Radical feminism, however, remains the one perspective least understood by most nurses, perhaps because it does not offer an immediate resolution to the problem of women's oppression.

A FEMINIST UTOPIAN WORLD OF CARING

First, war has been outlawed by world leaders—the majority of whom are women. Defense spending has been converted to "peace spending" to provide adequate food, housing, employment, and health care. Cooperative instead of competitive modes regulate world trade. National governments have disappeared along with nuclear energy. The United Nations decides on policy geared toward a fair distribution of the world's resources.

Caring has been *socialized*. Caring at all levels—be it child care, illness care, or elderly care is viewed as a societal responsibility. Caring here becomes the highest ethical concern of being human. Women and men inclined to practice caring professionally choose to be care workers with good pay and high status. Gender and class problems fade away to allow nurses to have the kind of caring relationship with clients described by Leininger (1984), Watson (1979, 1985, 1987), Noddings (1984), and others. Such a professional goal attains broad societal support.

All women or men doing caring work in their private lives, as described by Graham (1983) and Sommers and Shields (1987), are paid and given broad-based institutionalized sources of help avoiding the social isolation, fragmented work careers, and financial sacrifices that face such people today. For example, many nurses are doing "caring work" in their private as well as their professional lives leaving little time or space for their own needs. The *socialization* of caring work, particularly with our aging population, is an utopian idea whose time has come.

BACK TO REALITY

Since utopia must wait, what can be done now to enhance nurses' ability to care? Several alternatives are available:

- First, we can support a national health care plan (NHCP) that would provide all citizens with access to nursing. As we give this support we must be careful to not allow medicine to continue its dominance over nursing. We must also demand reimbursement for autonomous nursing care.

- Collective bargaining can be used by practicing nurses to insist on working conditions that allow them to have caring relationships with patients and to have appropriate pay for their caring work.
- Nurses can conduct clinical research on the importance of caring on patient outcomes and disseminate the findings in lay, public health, medical, and nursing literature.
- Women's studies offer feminist theories and their application to a multitude of women's issues such as the nature of women's work, caring and nursing.
- Faculty developing nursing curricula, at all levels, can draw on feminist theories and research methods.

Nursing can no longer afford to ignore feminist theory and the insights that it can provide about our ability to care. As Jo Ann Ashley (1980) stated:

Women nurses are women first. If we consistently remember this, accepting our heritage and strengths as women, our politics of care can begin. (p. 21)

REFERENCES

Andrist, L. (1988). A feminist framework for graduate education in women's health. *Journal of Nursing Education, 27*(2), 66–70.

Arms, S. (1975). *Immaculate desception: A new look at women and children in America.* Boston: Houghton Mifflin.

Ashley, J. A. (1980). Power in structured misogny: Implications for the politics of care. *Advances in Nursing Science, 2*(3), 3–22.

Ashley, J. (1976). *Hospitals paternalism and the role of the nurse.* New York: Teachers College Press.

Barry, K. (1979). *Female sexual slavery* (2nd ed.). New York: New York University Press.

Bartky, S. (1977). Toward a phenomenology of feminist consciousness. In M. Vetterling-Braggin, F. Ellison, & J. English (Eds.), *Feminism and philosophy.* Totawa, N J: Littlefield, Adams & Co.

Belenky, M., Clinchy, B., Goldberger, N., & Tarule, J. (1986). *Women's ways of knowing: The development of self, voice and mind.* New York: Basic Books.

Bockman, D. (1988). *Nurturing the human spirit in the work place: Caring for the nurse.* Unpublished paper presented at the Tenth National Research Care Conference, Boca Raton, Florida May 1–3.

Boulding, E. (1976). *The underside of history: A view of women through time.* Boulder, CO: Westview Press.

Bowles, G., & Duelli Klein, R. (Eds.). (1983). *Theories of women's studies.* Boston: Routledge & Kegan Paul.

Braverman, H. (1974). *Labor and monopoly capital: The degradation of work in the twentieth century.* New York: Monthly Review of Books.

Bunch, C., & Pollock, S. (1983). *Learning our way: Essays in feminist education.* Trumansburg, NY: The Crossing Press.

Chesler, P. (1972). *Women and madness.* New York: Avon Books.

Chinn, P., Wheeler, C., Ray, A., & Wheeler, E. (1987, November). Just between friends. *American Journal of Nursing,* 1456–1458.

Chinn, P., & Wheeler, C. (1985). Feminism and nursing: Can nursing afford to remain aloof from the women's movement? *Nursing Outlook, 33*(2), 74–77.

Connors, D. (1980). Sickness unto death: Medicine as mythic, necrophilic and Iatrogenic. *Advances in Nursing Science, 2*(3), 39–51.

Daly, M. (1978). *Gyn/Ecology: The metaethics of radical feminism.* Boston: Beacon Press.

Dodson, G. E. (1982). *Patriarchy as a conceptual trap.* Wellesley, MA: Roundtable Press.

Eisenstein, Z. (1979). *Capitalist patriarchy and the case for socialist feminism.* New York: Monthly Review Press.

Fee, E. (1983). Women and health care: A comparison of theories. In E. Fee (Ed.), *Women and health: The politics of sex in medicine.* Farmingdale, NY: Baywood Publishing Co.

Ferguson, K. (1984). *The feminist case against bureaucracy.* Philadelphia: Temple University Press.

Finch, J., Groves, D. (Eds.). (1983). *A labour of love: women, work and caring.* Boston: Routledge & Kegan Paul.

French, M. (1985). *Beyond power: On women, men and morals.* New York: Summit Books.

Friedan, B. (1963). *The feminine mystique*. New York: Norton.

Fry, S. (19   ) Ethic of caring: Can it survive in nursing? *Nursing Outlook, 36*(1), 48.

Gaut, D. (1984). A philosophic orientation to caring research. In M. Leininger (Ed.), *Care, the essence of nursing and health*. Thorofare, NJ: Slack.

Gilligan, C. (1982). *In a different voice*. Cambridge: Harvard University Press.

Graham, H. (1983). A labour of love. In J. Finch & D. Groves (Eds.). *A labour of love: Women, work and caring*. Boston: Routledge & Kegan Paul.

Greenleaf, N. P. (1980). Sex-segregated occupations: Relevance for nursing. *Advances in Nursing Science, 2*(3), 23–37.

Greenleaf, N. P. *Leadership without power: Contradictions faced by nurse executives in the American health industry*. Unpublished manuscript.

Heide, W. S. (1985). *Feminism for the health of it*. Buffalo: Margaretdaughters, Inc.

Jagger, A. M., & Rothenberg, P. S. (Eds.). (1984). *Feminist frameworks: Alternatives theoretical accounts of the relations between women and men* (2nd ed.). New York: McGraw-Hill.

Jagger, A. (1983). *Feminist politics and human nature*. Totowa, NJ: Rowman & Allanheld.

King, Y. (1988, February). Coming of age with the greens. *Zeta Magazine*, 16–19.

Krysl, M., & Watson, J. (1988). Existential moments of caring: Facets of nursing and social support. *Advances in Nursing Science, 10*(2), 12–17.

Kushner, R. (1975). *Breast cancer: A personal history and investigative report*. New York: Harcourt, Brace, Jovanovich.

Leininger, M. (1984). *Care: The essence of nursing and health*. Thorofare, NJ: Slack.

Leininger, M. (1978). *Transcultural nursing: Concepts, theories and practices*. New York: John Wiley & Sons.

Lovell, M. (1980). The politics of medical deception: Challenging the trajectory of history. *Advances in Nursing Science, 2*, 73–86.

Lowe, M., & Hubbard, R. (Eds.). (1983). *Woman's nature: Rationalization's of inequality*. New York: Pergamon Press.

MacPherson, K. I. (1987). Osteoporosis: The new flaw in woman or in science? *Health Values, 11*(4), 57–62.

MacPherson, K. I. (1985). Osteoporosis and menopause: A feminist analysis of the social construction of a syndrome. *Advances in Nursing Science, 7*(4), 11–22.

MacPherson, K. (1983). Feminist methods: A new paradigm for nursing research. *Advances in Nursing Science, 5*(2), 17–24.

MacPherson, K. (1981). Menopause as disease: The social construction of a metaphore. *Advances in Nursing Science, 3*(2), 95–113.

Melosh, B. (1982). *The physicians hand: Work culture and conflict in American nursing.* Philadelphia: Temple University.

Mishler, E. G. (1979). Meaning in context. Is there any other kind? *Harvard Educational Review, 49*(2), 1–19.

Moccia, P. (1988). At the faultline: Social activism and caring. *Nursing Outlook, 36*(1), 30–33.

Moccia, P. (1987, June). The nature of the nursing shortage: Will crisis become structure? *Nursing & Health Care,* 321–322.

Moccia, P. (1986, October). Are we dying for nuclear weapons? *American Journal of Nursing,* 1124–1125.

Morgan, S. (1986). *Coping with hysterectomy: Your own choice, your own solutions.* New York: New American Library.

Nightingale, F. (1860). *Notes on Nursing: What it is and what it is not.* London: Harrison.

Noddings, N. (1984). *Caring: A feminine approach to ethics and moral education.* Los Angeles: University of California Press.

Peplau, H. (1952). *Interpersonal relations in nursing: A conceptual frame of reference for psychodynamic nursing.* New York: Putnam.

Ray, M. (1984). The development of a classification system of institutional caring. In M. Leininger (Ed.), *Care, the essence of nursing and health.* Thorofare, NJ: Slack Inc.

Raymond, J. (1986). *A passion for friends: Toward a philosophy of female affection.* Boston: Beacon Press.

Reinharz, S. (1979). *On becoming a social scientist: From survey research and participant observation to experiential.* San Francisco: Jossey-Bass, Inc.

Reinharz, S., Bombyk, M., & Wright, J. (1983). Methodological issues in feminist research: A bibliography of literature in women's studies, sociology and psychology. *Women's Studies International Forum, 6*(4), 437–454.

Reverby, S. (1987). *Ordered to care: The dilemma of American nursing.* New York: Cambridge University Press.

Roberts, H. (Ed.) (1981). *Doing feminist research.* Boston: Routledge & Kegan Paul.

Salmon, J. (1987). The medical profession and the corporatization of the health sector. *Theoretical Medicine, 8,* 19–29.

Sayers, J. (1982). *Biological politics: Feminist and anti-feminist perspectives.* New York: Tavistock.

Seaman, B., & Seaman, G. (1977). *Women and the crisis in sex hormones.* New York: Bantam Books.

Sheston, M. (1988, May). *Caring in nursing education: The development of a construct.* Unpublished paper presented at the Tenth National Research Care Conference, Boca Raton, Florida.

Sommers, T., & Shields, L. (Eds.). (1987). *Women take care: The consequences of caregiving in today's society.* Gainesville, FL: Triad Publishing.

Stanley, L., & Wise, S. (1983). *Breaking out: Feminist consciousness and feminist research.* Boston: Routledge & Kegan Paul.

Thompson, J. L. (1990). *Exploring myth and symbol with refugee women: An application of feminist archetypal theory.* Unpublished manuscript.

Thompson, J. L. (1985). Practical discourse in nursing: Going beyond empiricism and historicism. *Advances in Nursing Science, 7*(4), 59–71.

Thompson, J. L. (1987). Critical scholarship: The critique of domination in nursing. *Advances in Nursing Science, 10*(1), 27–38.

Vetterling-Graggin, M., Elliston, F., & English, J. (1977). *Feminism and philosophy.* Totowa, NJ: Littlefield, Adams & Co.

Voda, A., Dinnerstein, M., & O'Donnell, S. (1982). *Changing perspectives on menopause.* Austin: University of Texas Press.

Watson, J. (1979). *Nursing: The philosophy and science of caring.* Boston: Little, Brown and Company.

Watson, J. (1985). *Nursing: Human science and Human Care.* Norwalk, CT: Appleton-Century-Crofts.

Watson, J. (1987). Nursing on the caring edge: Metaphorical vignettes. *Advances in Nursing Science, 10*(1), 10–18.

Wolf, K. A. (1980). ANS open forum. *Advances in Nursing Science, 2*(3), 99.

4

A Study of Nursing's Feminist Ideology

Karen L. Miller

The late nurse historian, Teresa Christy (1971), was fond of saying, both in writing and in her public speeches, that it was "unfortunate" that nurses as professional women did not follow the example set by some of our early leaders to fight for equality for women. Unlike Lavinia Dock, Adelaide Nutting, Lillian Wald, Annie Goodrich and others of their time, nurses did not then and have not since taken an active lead in the women's movement.

As JoAnn Ashley (1975) might reiterate, were she here today, "to the detriment of our own growth as professional persons, we nurses are among the most conservative of the conservatives. With rare exceptions, we have been nonfeminists. This failure may lead to nursing's inability to liberate both education and practice in our society" (p. 68).

While it remains true that nurses are not rushing to join the ranks of radical feminists in their quest for equality in all social spheres, it seems to me that in the recent past claims have been made by nurse scholars (e.g., Benoliel, 1975; MacPherson, 1983; Jacobs & Chinn, 1987; Thompson, 1985; and Chinn & Wheeler, 1985) that nursing is most appropriately considered in the context of gender-based roles and feminist theory.

At the 1987 Western Society for Research in Nursing Conference, Jacobs and Chinn (1987) presented a model of nursing knowledge that extended the work of Carper (1978) on "ways of knowing" for nursing. Problems of language and meaning inherent in nursing's knowledge base were discussed with emphasis on nursing choices influenced by empirics, ethics, esthetics, and the personal. At this same meeting, Watson (1987) presented the popular book, *Women's Ways of Knowing*, by Belenky et al. (1986) as theoretically parallel to the evolution of nursing's human science approach to knowledge development. Certainly, these presentations attest to the interest of nurse scholars in feminist ideas about the personal and alternative ways of perceiving the world, at least the world as it is for working nurses.

If claims such as these are justified, the relationship between feminism and nursing must be explicated in order to clarify the potential of feminist perspective for knowledge generation in the discipline. The study that I engaged in and present here evolved from a critical science orientation to the exploration of this relationship. I wanted to establish a theoretically adequate description of feminist ideology relative to nursing that would allow us to incorporate feminist ideas in an organized way as a basis for research and that would move us forward in our appreciation of feminism as a means of social and intellectual change. (Had I realized the breadth of such a task, I might not have set out on this challenge!)

Nevertheless, I began the research utilizing a foundational inquiry design. This type of design is intended for the pursuit of unique interpretations of phenomena within the context of a specific discipline. Its nature is philosophical and hermeneutical. It was described by Smith (1983) in her book, *The Idea of Health*, as "a semantic investigation or an examination of the meaning of the written word" (p. 251). Foundational inquiry procedes from questions that reveal ambiguity, discrepancy, problematic definition, or that lack sufficient clarity (Smith, 1986). The phenomenon of feminist ideology as it relates to nursing lacks clarity in the nursing literature. Yet, as a discipline, we have become increasingly interested in preserving nursing's feminine values and heritage as a women's profession.

Consideration of feminist ideology and theory as foundationsal to nursing science was predicated on two fundamental assumptions:

1. The nursing profession is predominantly female (98 percent) and is socioculturally perceived as "feminine."

2. The essential work of nurses in human caring involves a feminine, service-oriented, humanistic, and nurturing role.

The central thesis of this study was that feminist ideology is foundational to the discipline of nursing and the domain of nursing administration.

DESIGN AND METHODOLOGY

The investigation included conceptual, literary content, and ethnographic analysis of historical and contemporary feminists and feminism in nursing literature. The content selection process identified those literary pieces most representative of feminist intellecutal development and the relationship of feminist thought to nursing's theoretical evolution. More than 200 literary references resulted from computerized and manual sampling of the literature of a variety of disciplines. This anthology provided the database for the study.

Analysis was accomplished through the use of two computer analysis programs: (1) a "flat" database categorization system, designed for large volume information access and search capabilities and (2) the "Ethnograph" (Seidel, Kjolseth, & Clark, 1985) computer tool which is designed for analysis of text-based data. The qualitative coding mechanisms required for both of these computerized analyses led to deductive conceptual interpretation of the feminist and nursing and feminism literature.

The data was analyzed in two separate stages or volumes:

1. Evolution of feminist theory.
2. Contemporary feminist ideology.

Each of these stages comprised historical information which was categorized by typologies based on theoretical stance as well as chronology. For instance, I used five philosophically distinct viewpoints as a basis for evaluating the history of feminist theory, and then two chronological periods to look at feminist theory development in the last 28 years. (I must add that this part of the research was a wonderful adventure in history and women's literature. The process of learning another field was quite time-consuming, but it was so gratifying to become familiar with the writings of "significant sisters" in our history. I'm sure many of the other presenters have had similar experiences.)

RESULTS

While the results of this study represent contextual (or within the discipline of nursing) interpretations of the literature database, one difficulty in analysis was the semantic confusion in definition of the phenomenon under study. Both the feminist and nursing and feminism literature presented various definitions of feminism, feminist theory, and ideology that needed clarification. Historically, nursing has not embraced feminism as a philosophy or set of activities, in part due to its ambiguous and socially constructed definitions.

Definitions of feminism describe a variety of perspectives or "points of view" of both women and men who express a distinctly feminine or nontraditional way of viewing life experiences. Mitchell and Oakley (1986) maintain that "feminism takes its meaning from the moment," that it is capable of incorporating and adapting to environmental influences. There is a significant dimension of flexibility in this phenomenon. Stanley and Wise (1983) define feminism in a way that is useful for interpretations of nursing phenomena. "Feminism is a set of beliefs and a set of theoretical constructions about the nature of women's social reality" (p. 55). As a "set of beliefs," feminist ideology may be interpreted as a social movement to activate these beliefs. As a "set of theoretical constructions," feminist ideology provides the basis for interpretation and reorganization of social reality.

A feminist is one who advocates for women the same rights that society accords men, particularly in the spheres of economics and politics. In this sense, feminism is not totally gender specific. Despite controversy in the feminist literature, I believe that men may be feminists, in fact, many are. By the same token, not all women are feminists or support feminist beliefs.

Similar to nursing theory, feminist theory is "action oriented," used for explanation and as a guide for research. The diversity of definitions of feminism and of feminist theory is built on a shared perception that feminist perspective deserves to be considered—that "difference" makes a difference!

The label, *feminist ideology*, was chosen for this investigation to allow a broad conceptualization of feminist perspective, thought, ideas, and theory that may influence the discipline of nursing generally and the domain of nursing administration specifically.

Taking the various definitions of feminist phenomena into account, this study was undergirded by an assumption of generization. Historical and present attempts to define feminism and feminist theory imply that the world is *genderized*—socially and intellectually differentiated by sex. This crucial assumption was clearly substantiated in the data. For example, ethicist Nel Noddings (1987) writes that genderization is a "fact-of life" in the historical development of philosophy. She argues that basic Western philosophic thought has been mistakenly construed as gender free, lacking sexual bias, when, in fact, bias can be easily estrapolated from classic philosophic literature. Other feminist and nursing scholars make similar cases for genderization in their disciplines.

Analysis of the literature data for insights into the relationship of feminist ideology to nursing revealed a wide variety of feminist intellectual and social issues of potential interest to our discipline. Response to the research questions took essentially two directions:

1. Delineation of perspectives on nursing and feminism that emerged from computer analysis of text.

2. Identification of central themes which "bind" feminism and nursing together intellectually and socially in specific ways.

First, the following three analytical perspectives for evaluating feminist ideology and nursing resulted:

1. Nurses as a Workforce

2. Nursing as a Profession of Women

3. Nursing as a Scientific Discipline

Each of these perspectives was analyzed in terms of literary support references written by feminists and by nurses. The perspectives were then identified through the coding and categorization processes.

Nurses as a Workforce

Work and labor issues are major concerns for the nursing profession. Feminist ideological perspectives on women's work offer nursing ways to evaluate these issues which are heavily related to nursing's sociocultural status as a "feminine" profession. At its worst, feminist literature on work and labor issues refers to nursing as part of a group of female-predominant occupations termed "the female job ghetto" (Ferree & Hess, 1985, p. 144). Nursing, more often than not, is portrayed by feminists as an occupation, not a profession. It is an example of a family or "household" task shifted to the "outside world" of production. As women were never financially rewarded for the service aspects of domestic life, so, too, are they economically unrewarded for similar work in capitalist society. These views emanate from the socialist/Marxist feminist viewpoint. From this perspective, one might argue that the difficulties nurses have in receiving salaries comensurate with their education and expertise is due to a much larger societal issue than to a simple problem of employment.

The relationship between the occupation of nursing and the historical, social evolution of women is clearly evident in the nursing and feminism literature. Part of nursing's difficulty in resolving the issues involved with viewing "nurses as a workforce" is that nursing perceives itself to be a profession which emphasizes individual nurse accountability for practice. Virginia Cleland (1981, p. 17) writes that the professional role of the nurse, to care for patients, seems in opposition to labor issues focusing on the "condition of working" as a nurse. The nursing literature indicates that nurses' identification with "labor" versus "professional" worker is still devisive for nurses.

Nursing as a Profession of Women

While most direct feminist comment on nursing is related to work and labor issues, evaluation of the second perspective incorporated both liberal and cultural feminist orientations. These emphasize feminine qualities and characteristics, holistic vision, natural rights of women, the power of women and female intellect and reasoning abilities. The data support the belief that nursing is presently immersed in a search for expressions of nursing's reality and ways of articulating the meaning of subjective experiences with patients, families, other health care providers, systems, and among nurses themselves. Our literature indicates that we are in the process of building our own collective consciousness-raising about ourselves as nurses in a female-predominant profession. We seem to be moving toward a stronger sense of community and colleagueship whereby nurses are learning how to network and consult each other, and to use each other's special knowledge as manager, caregiver, and educator.

This sense of community is allowing us a more positive integration of men into the profession, appreciating their differences while acknowledging their unique contributions—just as we are coming to terms with the feminine in nursing.

Nursing as a Scientific Discipline

Since the focus of this research was on feminist and nursing intellectual congruence, the majority of literature emphasized the third perspective. It is obvious that our discipline is in a transition toward acceptance of a wider range of viewpoints on science, including epistemological alternatives. In the sense that feminist study is a discipline, nursing seems to be taking on feminist disciplinary beliefs and actions. Some of the presentations at this conference will address aspects of feminist science as they relate to nursing, such as feminist perspectives in research design and feminist science in the profession of nursing. Our ties to feminist, or at least alternative, approaches to science are becoming stronger and better articulated.

CONCEPTUAL THEMES

As the study evolved, the ethnographic content analysis revealed several conceptual themes that described specific feminist ideological tenets which enhance our understanding of nursing practice, research, and theory development. The themes were not evident in each literature piece, but emerged through analysis of the literature composite. Taken together, these themes form the basis of "nursing's feminist ideology" as conceived in this study.

The Personal is Political

A slogan of feminism and politics, "the personal as political," argues that personal and intimate experience is not isolated, individual, or undetermined, but rather is social, political, and systematic (Kramarae & Treichler, 1985). Personal experience as inherent to public life is central to feminist ideology and highly relevant to professional nursing. This theme emphasizes the importance of the subjective, and rejects traditional insistence that the objective and structural are fundamentally separate from the personal. Traditional, patriarchal standards are apparent in the health care arena where personal investment in professional work has been historically undervalued. Unfortunately, this stance has placed nursing in a particularly difficult position: as clinicians we value objective, prescriptive, technical actions in health care delivery, and as caregivers we are committed to the personal in caring as the essence of our work. Nursing is a personal, caring commitment in a public domain. As such, it becomes imperative that we find ways to make the political more personal.

Invisibility

The feminist concept of invisibility refers to the virtual absence of women's words and activities from classic literature and history. Besides women's historical invisibility as a factor for nursing as a female-predominant profession, lack of women's visibility has contributed to the undervaluing of care as part of socially assigned "women's work." Colliere (1985) urges nurses to become more aware of their sociocultural invisibility in order to have a better understanding of problems in health care where our work is not always recognized as essential.

Marginality

Marginality exists when an individual lives in two worlds simultaneously, one of which, by prevailing stands, is regarded as superior (Duelli Klein, 1983). Feminist ideology holds that marginal persons in society are those whose roles threaten those in power. Marginals live at the edge of what is socially acceptable and culturally normal. Feminists use this term to describe the place of women in society. The notion of marginality is especially significant for conceptualizing the status of professional nursing. Nurses are marginal by virtue of their work, as well as by gender. What occurs as a result of nursing's marginal status is development of care modalities that are unspoken, unrecognized, and unappreciated by the dominant groups and, therefore, by society at large.

Feminist Consciousness

It is clear that some nurse scholars consider gender-based conceptualizations of reality as essential to the discipline of nursing. Nurses are searching for ways of expressing reality as understood and experienced by women professionals in health care delivery systems. It seems that this search is moving toward feminist consciousness as a legitimate way of understanding reality. This aspect of feminist ideology recognizes historical and present ways of thinking about and perceiving our world that have emanated from feminine life experiences as separate and distinct from traditionally recognized, masculine experiences—those which dominate social orientation to health care.

Diverse Representations of Members

Another emergent theme is the idea of diverse representation. There was no definitive definition of feminism and many interpretations of the term or group were available, depending on perspective. Nursing, too, has many representations and lacks clear definition. This historical image confusion about the role of the nurse translates into a lack of specific social expectations for nursing education, practice, and scholarship.

Paradoxical Goals

Both feminism and nursing have been involved in attempts to establish the directions of their disciplines. For feminism the paradox lies in developmental goals: Are the goals of feminist scholarship to increase an awareness of alternative perspectives based on women's experiences or to work toward a social world that is not divided by gender roles? This paradox remains unsolved and has caused some alienation among feminist academicians and activists. A similar "paradox of goals" is evident in the discipline of nursing: While nurse scholars strive to develop a strong theoretical base of nursing knowledge which emphasizes individual professionalism and autonomy in practice, there is a strong political drive among nurses to increase nursing's public identification as a labor force with group power and solidarity.

Theory Building as an On-going Process

This study supports the contention that both feminist theorists and nursing theorists have encountered similar problems in theory development, particularly in disseminating theoretical ideas to those outside the discipline. In effect, both feminists and nurses face patriarchal bias. In the health care industry, recognition of nursing's theoretical contribution is often diminished by consideration of nursing as an employee group engaging in practice that does not require a specialized knowledge base. Feminists believe that this kind of traditional discrimination serves to lessen the threat of women's social and professional contributions to those in power. Both feminist and nurse scholars are committed to theory building as a means for organizing the thoughts and ideas of their disciplines toward future goals.

Division Between Leadership and Constituency

A problem basic to nursing administration practice is the perceived division between the leadership group in nursing, including educators and executives, and the nurses who "do the work" of nursing. This same issue is a problem for the feminist movement. During recent years, feminists have been concerned about alienation of women from the movement. Likewise, nurse administrators are concerned that practicing nurses do not relate well to nursing leaders and academic nursing issues. Those activities which are necessary for the evolution of the discipline seem distant from the highly technical and crisis-oriented world of the working nurse (Biordi, 1986).

These eight central and binding themes are specific feminist tenets that are closely related to intellectual themes in nursing's evolutionary development as a discipline. In our historical, intellectual traditions of holism and conservatism, nurses have not formally integrated the positive, enhancing aspects of feminist ideology. This ideology evolves from women's experience in the world as separate from traditional, male experience. Such an ideological base is shared by the nursing profession by virtue of its historical existence as female-predominant and by virtue of its social recognition as a feminine occupation. Unlike other female-predominant professions, we have experienced a theoretical, if not political, congruence with the intellectual traditions of feminism. This congruence can be validated through analyses of the feminist and nursing literature. This study identified eight congruent intellectual themes which specifically describe feminist ideology in nursing, along with some consistent theoretical strands which can be traced through historical literature sources.

The face-value criticism of this analysis is that the investigation is inherently divisive and dualistic in nature. Such an approach may promote gender-based separation among nurses and conceptualizations of the nursing role and patient care. I do not totally deny this criticism. However, my belief, strongly substantiated by this research, is that if we as nurses are to fully explore our theoretical and praxicological development, we must first explore our socio-cultural position as a female-dominant profession. Certainly, none of us were educated as undergrads from this perspective!

Analysis of feminist ideology provides us useful insights about female consciousness which is at the core of nursing. Our goal is intellectual "holism" as a concept descriptive of our discipline. This goal is congruent with feminist intellecutal traditions. It behooves us to search for our intellectual roots as the logical starting place for research and theory generation. The dualism of this search will fade as we incorporate this new knowledge and establish a stronger nursing identity in the world. The inclusion of feminist ideology as foundational to nursing implies its significance for research and theory generation in our discipline.

SYNTHESIS THEORY

The final phase of this research project was to incorporate the central and binding themes into existing nursing practice frameworks. I used an original model of nursing administration practice and theory development that I had designed earlier. This framework evolved from Meleis' (1985) ideas on theory building in nursing. The process of placing the themes within the context of nursing administration led to the development of a *synthesis theory*, which states: *the practice roles of advocacy, consciousness raising, and empowerment in nursing administration synthesize feminist ideological themes central to nursing.* The model conveys both the process of nursing administration and the specific practice roles that bring together concepts of feminist ideology relative to this domain. Such a synthesis guides actions as well as research and theory construction. The following example illustrates this concept.

The *advocacy role* of the nurse administrator is an extension of the basic role of the nurse as patient advocate. It is fundamental advocacy based on the nature of the nurse-patient relationship, our common humanity, needs, and rights (Curtain, 1986). Nurses advocate for, represent or speak for the patient. We view ourselves as responsible for the needs and rights of patients and families in various health care systems. Gadow (1984) refers to advocacy as a form of caring, part of nursing's unique contribution to the psychological and physiological health of our clients. Administrative advocacy requires constant awareness of the situation of nurses within the health care environment and a sensitivity to their needs and rights as professionals.

The need for administrative advocacy arises in consideration of the feminist notion of *marginality* in nursing. Marginal status implies social position outside prevailing standards, such as the position of nurses in patriarchal health care systems. As a result of nursing's marginality, the caring acts of nurses are not often recognized nor are they appreciated by the dominant groups in health care (Ashley, 1976). Nurse administrators can take the initiative to decrease the marginal status of nurses for whom they advocate. By informing nurses clearly and often about their many contributions to the care of clients and by representing nurses in a positive, constructive way to others in the health care industry, administrators can publicize the worth of nurse. Executives have the opportunity to enhance nurses' self-appreciation and to bring an understanding of the value of nursing to other professionals.

Consciousness raising is an action designed to incorporate personal experience and subjective perception into ways of thinking, understanding reality, and personal decision making (Costain, 1981). While nurses work in a highly interpersonal environment with patients, we have evolved our perceptions of reality from traditional, patriarchal models of science and health care delivery. As a female-predominant profession, nursing must learn more about its roots in women's experiences. We must learn how to include these experiences openly in practice for the benefit of clients. By virtue of her leadership and authority position, the nurse administrator can lead the way in concerted efforts to recognize *feminist consciousness* as a valuable addition to nursing "ways of thinking." This role requires an awareness of one's philosophy of life and the ability to reflect on personal perceptions of work situations. It means that the administrator must accept herself and her own contributions, as well as the personal limitations we all experience. She must be able to articulate the importance of feminine, subjective knowledge to nurses with whom she communicates.

The *empowerment* role of the nurse executive is in opposition to the traditional conceptualization of power as dominance. Power and control for the purpose of dominating another or a group is the primary value in our political world (French, 1985). Feminists believe that dominance and control are the natural underpinnings of oppression and lead to essential human separation. The concept of empowerment is relational in nature. It implies affirmation of the self and others, without loss of personal control and independence. Traditional views in health care support separation of personal experience from professional work—isolation of the self in interactions. Feminist ideology disavows such separation. The "personal is political" stance of feminism argues that personal experience is social and political. The empowering executive incorporates this "personal is political" alternative viewpoint. She promotes interactional relationships that affirm rather than overpower. Our commitment to human caring requires altruistic attention to the individual autonomy and rights of patients and families as part of the politics of health care.

CONCLUSION

Through these examples I have shown how feminist ideological tenets can be synthesized into domains of nursing—for present actions and future research. It is important that we act on our ideas, and that we not continue in our quiet, conservative mode of nursing behavior.

To understand the connection between feminism and nursing is to grasp a part of nursing's heritage and intellectual constitution that has been present, but unexplored, in our profession. The analyses that resulted from this research are a beginning attempt to delineate this relationship. I believe that if we are to survive as a clinical discipline in future health care systems, we must interpret ourselves within the context of both past and present socioeconomic environments. This means in part that we must recognize the "feminine" in what we have been, in what we are, the limitations of our past, and the potential strength of a future founded upon feminist thought.

REFERENCES

Ashley, J. (1975, September). Nursing and early American feminism. *American Journal of Nursing*, 68–70.

Ashley, A. (1976). *Hospitals, paternalism and the role of the nurse.* New York: Teachers College Press, Columbia University.

Belenky, M., Clinchy, B., Goldberger, N., & Tarule, J. (1986). *Women's ways of knowing.* New York: Basic Books.

Benoliel, J. (1975). Scholarship—a woman's perspective. *Image, 7*(2), 22–27.

Biordi, D. (1986). Nursing service administrators: Marginality and the public person. *Nursing Clinics of North America, 21*(1), 173–183.

Carper, B. (1978). Fundamental patterns of knowing in nursing. *Advances in Nursing Science, 1*(1), 13–23.

Chinn, P., & Wheeler, C. (1985). Feminism and nursing. *Nursing Research, 33*(2), 74–77.

Christy, T. (1971, February). Equal rights for women: Voices from the past. *American Journal of Nursing*, 62–67.

Cleland, V. (1981, July). Taft-Hartley amended: Implication for nursing—the professional model. *Journal of Nursing Administration*, 17–21.

Colliere, M. (1986). Invisible care and invisible women as health care-providers. *International Journal of Nursing Studies, 23*(2), 99–112.

Costain, A. (1981). Representing women: The transition from social movement to interest groups. *Western Political Quarterly, 34,* 100–113.

Curtain, L. (1986). The nurse as advocate. In E. Hein & J. Nicholoson (Eds.), *Contemporary leadership behavior: Selected readings* (pp. 129–136). Boston: Little, Brown.

Duelli Klein, R. (1983). How to do what we want to do: Thoughts about feminist methodology. In G. Bowles & R. Duelli Klein (Eds.), *Theories of women's studies* (pp. 88–104). New York: Routledge & Kegan Paul.

Ferree, M., & Hess, B. (1985). *Controversy and coalition: The new feminist movement.* Boston: Twayne.

French, M. (1985). *Beyond power: On women, men and morals.* New York: Ballantine Books.

Gadow, S. (1984, March). Existential advocacy as a form of caring: Technology, truth and touch. *Research seminar series: The development of nursing as a human science.* Denver, CO: University of Colorado Health Sciences Center.

Jacobs, M., & Chinn, P. (1987). The whole of knowing: A model of nursing knowledge. *Proceedings of the Western Society for Research in Nursing Conference, 20.* Boulder, CO: Western Institute of Nursing.

Kramarae, C., & Treichler, P. (1985). *A feminist dictionary.* Boston: Pandora Press.

MacPherson, K. (1983). Feminist methods: A new paradigm for nursing research. *Advances in Nursing Science, 5*(2), 17–25.

Meleis, A. (1985). *Theoretical nursing: Development and progress.* Philadelphia: J.B. Lippincott.

Mitchell, J., & Oakley, A. (1986). *What is feminism—a re-examination.* New York: Pantheon Books.

Noddings, N. (1987). Ethics from the standpoint of women. In D. Rhodes (Ed.), *Theoretical perspectives on sexual difference.*

Seidel, J., Kjolseth, R., & Clark, J. (1985). *The ethnograph.* Littleton, CO: Qualis Research.

Smith, J. (1983). *The idea of health.* New York: Teacher's College Press, Columbia University.

Smith, J. (1986). The idea of health: Doing foundational inquiry. In P. Munhall & C. Oiler (Ed.), *Nursing research, a qualitative perspective* (pp. 250–261). Norwalk, CT: Appleton-Century-Crofts.

Stanley, L., & Wise, S. (1983). *Breaking out: Feminist consciousness and feminist research.* London: Routledge & Kegan Paul.

Thompson, J. (1985). Practical discourse in nursing: Going beyond empiricism and historicism. *Advances in Nursing Science, 7*(4), 59–71.

Watson, J. (1987). Advancing the art and science of human caring. In *Proceedings of the Western Society for Research in Nursing Conference, 20,* Boulder, CO: Western Institute of Nursing.

5

Researching the Lives of Eminent Women in Nursing: Rozella M. Schlotfeldt

Elizabeth R. Berrey

My paper contains echoes of ideas expressed by Dr.'s Boulding and Miller from this morning. Some of those echoes are harmonious. Others are distinctly dissonant because, like some of you, I am in sharp disagreement with portions of this morning's presentation. How can this be? How is it that we find ourselves so conflicted? First, many of us as women have, unfortunately, tended to believe the noise pollution (Raymond, 1982) from the dominant culture about ourselves as women and our profession. However, I am here to affirm that we come from a long line of women of determination and persistence, of passion, of intellect, and of courage—our foresisters in nursing. And perhaps the best explanation for the incongruent and controversial perspectives we've heard on definitions of feminism—that is, the roles of those women who are for and with women contrasted with those women who are for and with men (see Raymond regarding: "heterorelational privilege")—and feminism vis-a-vis nursing are best captured in a statement that Dagmar Celeste [First Mate of Ohio] recently made: "Women are the only oppressed group that sleep with the enemy every night, so it's no wonder some of us get confused!"

My research is born out of my respect for, and love of, women, our profession, and a commitment to a feminist, woman-centered critique. It was designed to focus on the lives of eminent women in nursing so as to uncover their unique, experiential life features. A single narrator, one eminent nurse, was then selected to support the intent of the study.

Our society has been named an androcentric (or patriarchal) society by current feminist writers in the fields of philosophy (Callaway, 1981; Daly, 1978, 1984; Frye, 1983; Mahowald, 1983), sociology (Bernard, 1985), history (Cook, 1977; Raymond, 1982), theology (Christ & Plaskow, 1979; Daly, 1978; Kolbenschlag, 1979; Radford Ruether, 1983; Russell, 1976; Schussler Fiorenza, 1983; Wilson-Kastner, 1983), nursing (Ashley, 1980; Chinn, 1982; Chinn & Wheeler, 1985; Christy, 1971; Cleland, 1971) and politics (Atkinson, 1978; Friedan, 1970; Steinem, 1983). A consequence of living in an androcentric society is that women are oppressed. As a result, women's lives are obscured, trivialized (Bernard, 1985; Chinn & Wheeler, 1985; Cook, 1977) and seen as marginal to history (Schussler Fiorenza, 1983). Consequently, as a women's profession, much of the history of nursing overall is hidden, and women nurses as individuals are not visible within the historical context of this androcentric society as knowledgeable innovators in health care nor, as with other women, "people [with] . . . political and social power" (Friedan, 1970, p. 19). Furthermore, the androcentric scholarly paradigm has relegated research about women to the "periphery of scholarly concerns" (Schussler Fiorenza, 1983, p. 43)— insignificant, trivial, and unworthy of scholarly attention. At the same time, members of a profession are obligated to preserve and transmit their profession's heritage.

In the face of this androcentric proscription, there has not been a consistent commitment to research that which underlies the past and present circumstances in the nursing profession. As Irene Palmer (1986, p. 11) says, the profession lacks authoritative life histories of the "magnificent and visionary women who shaped health care and nursing." Nurses and the public are deprived of a perspective provided by a critical assessment of the ideas, ideals, and efforts of these women, as well as an understanding of the generative forces that gave rise to them. Comprehensive research into the lives of nursing leaders that goes beyond the published biographical vignettes, sketches, and comparisons is missing. Research of nursing's heritage is, then, a necessary foundation for nursing scholarship. Indeed, JoAnne Ashley (1976) said about nursing over a decade ago: "Our identity has suffered greatly because we have not carefully studied our history and incorporated historical knowledge into theoretical and clinical teachings. Without this knowledge, the foundations of nursing have indeed been shaky" (p. 29).

Gathering data to fill in the gaps of information about the lives of our nursing predecessors speaks to both the importance of accessing the unique, experiential features of these eminent nurses' lives and to the impact of an androcentric society on women's and nursing's heritage. Some women have made acclaimed contributions to nursing against great odds imposed by living, and by practicing their profession, in an oppressive society.

Nor has there been a study that explores the interactional, person-to-person relationship systems of nurse leaders. Because of the lack of such research, the sustaining networks of love and support that may exist (and have been shown to exist for other professionally and politically active women) go unrecognized in the lives of these nurses. In an androcentric society, such networks are critical to women's ability to "work in a hostile world where [they] are not in fact expected to survive" (Cook, 1977, p. 44).

In addition, the lives of individual human beings are seen on examination to be influenced by certain pervasive myths/beliefs which they inherit as part of their society's worldview. The power of these myths/beliefs to shape individual human lives is demonstrable. Therefore, if one is to discuss the complexity, wholeness, and fullness of a person—an individual life lived in the context of society, history, and family—it becomes necessary to consider the role of myths and symbols in human life.

Myths are illustrations or unexamined beliefs that inform human lives and, so doing, dictate human action. Persons live their lives, in part, by such myths. Those myths give meaning, substance, and unique definition to their lives. Myths can be viewed from three perspectives: societally generated myths, family/person generated myths, and myths handed down from ancient times. Some of these myths are collective societal myths (for example, that our society is free, moral, and just), or are idiosyncratic (that I am better than average, or doomed to fail). Family systems therapists such as Bowen (1978) theorize (and I use that term loosely and colloquially) that family members are controlled by family myths that are transmitted, over time, transgenerationally. There are also myths accumulated by human beings from ancient times. Myths are powerful and can be enhancing or limiting. Because of the pervasive androcentricity of our society, ancient myths have limiting, if not debilitating, effects on women's lives. However, identifying, naming, and critiquing myths are necessary for women to be free of them (Kolbenschlag, 1979).

In addition to being influenced by myths and beliefs, humans are also symbolic beings. Briefly, "symbols are representations for other things," and are used "to represent both concrete aspects of our world and abstract dimensions of our existence" (Wood, 1982, p. 6). A symbol may be a word, a gesture, or anything that represents an event, act, feeling, person, object, process, or relationship.

Human beings use symbols to define their immediate worlds and to define and create their futures and their pasts (Wood, 1982). Because of their symbolic ability, humans can transcend their immediate world, contemplate alternatives to it, and strive for better versions of themselves or their circumstances. Human beings can just as easily use symbols to restrict individual potential, diminish the value of their professions, and build barren relationships.

As Janeway (1971) says, "If there's nothing more powerful than an idea whose time has come, there is nothing more ubiquitously pervasive than an idea whose time won't go." The partition between men and women and their hierarchical ordering in the universe is so old and so built into our minds and our cultural background that it "produces an illusion of inevitability and revealed truth" (p. 7). As with other myths, the power of this myth is that it is understood as prescriptive rather that descriptive.

Social mythology is what society uses to cushion, manipulate, and explain (Janeway, 1971). For example, the ancient Chinese [men] concocted the principles of yang (male: active; interested in ideas and things) and yin (female: passive; interested in people and feelings). Yang and yin form a pattern, and patterns are pleasing. They endure over time because they offer a sense of control in a chaotic and confusing world. And no pattern is more central to the web of society and to an individual's life than the patterns of behavior constructed around sex differences. Thus, in this man's world, woman has her place. Because the myth is so powerful, women and men can live their lives, taking as true the social mythology given them. Hence, as in this study, a woman can give voice to "I'm a great admirer of medicine; it has everything I want," misperceiving that monopolizing the health care world was something achieved by medicine through hard work, education, determination, and commitment, not simply granted to medicine as its divine right, or as the natural order of things, which is the more accurate interpretation.

The consequences of this misperception are ravaging, particularly for women. For when all one's best efforts do *not* suffice, the women is subject to profound feelings of emptiness, which are filled up with harder work; with renewed efforts to identify with the male power structure, attempting to see with his eye, speak with his voice; with attempts to hide in shame one's identification with other women (if one even allows herself that any longer); or with attacks on other women so as to publicly disavow herself from her own kind and declare her allegiance to men. According to Frye (1983), the source of these (coerced) actions is

> *a mortal dread of being outside the field of vision of [Man's] eye. That eye gives all things meaning by connecting all things to each other by way of their references to one point —Man. We fear that if we are not in that web of meaning there will be no meaning: our work will be meaningless, our lives of no value, our accomplishments empty, our identities illusory. The reason for this dread . . . is that for most of*

us, including the exceptional, a woman existing outside the field of vision of man's arrogant eye is really inconceivable. (p. 80)

Again, the consequences of this misperception are ravaging. Not finding her own voice, the woman imitates male success patterns, erroneously believing that if she just does it right enough and long enough she can get there, too.

To do the research initially outlined, I formulated a synthesized morphogenic method that melded together compatible aspects of feminist critical hermeneutics, heuristic research, and the narration of live/oral history simply because one alone would not suffice.

As stated, the study purported to identify life themes and patterns in a living eminent women nurse that would fill in existing gaps of information about existential features of her life, describe themes and patterns that emerge from the influences of the historical climate as she perceived that climate, describe themes and patterns in her life that are reflected in, or have affected, her thinking about nursing as it developed over time, and contribute to change in the role and status of nursing by bringing new knowledge to light.

The narrator I selected was Rozella M. Schlotfeldt, an eminent nurse theorist, educator, *and* scholar in her early seventies. Dr. Schlotfeldt was encouraged to relate her life experience, in her own words, in response to four lead topics that I introduced: transgenerational family history, adult personal and professional relationship systems, perception of historical and cultural influences on her life, and development of earliest ideas about nursing up to the present.

There are three themes and five patterns that most clearly emerge in Rozella Schlotfeldt's thinking about nursing as it has evolved over time. Her essence in relationship to nursing is captured in her statement, "I just think that there is nobody more passionately involved in having nursing move toward what it could become. I always say what it could come, because it is not there [yet]."

Influenced by her mother, Rozella has been observing and thinking about nursing since her preschool days. As a young girl, she determined that she would be a nurse. Her early remembrances of her mother as a nurse were of a vigorous, hard-working, innovative, creative, "quite experimental," ambitious, determined, intelligent woman in great demand for the competent nursing care she rendered. Thus, Rozella left home, just past her seventeenth birthday, with this image of nursing clearly in view, to study at a research university that emphasized a strong liberalizing education for students of nursing.

Rozella began her academic career in nursing at the University of Colorado. From the University of Colorado to Wayne State University to Case Western Reserve University, Rozella Schlotfeldt was always an agent of change, often an innovator. It was at Case Western Reserve that Rozella made what she views as her most significant contributions, implementing them as a leader who believed in participative administration. Although Rozella was bound by her regard for authority and her identification with the male power structure, she was able to see beyond that and to develop her own style of administration that was intended to foster a mutual respectfulness. She was motivated by two awarenesses. First was her cognizance that she was "frightened, really frightened by the potential power of the deanship." She recalls, "I used to work overtime saying to myself, 'You have to listen, listen, listen, more than you talk . . . ' I used to work very hard to have [the faculty] make the decisions." Second was her belief that "human beings are striving, creative people," and, therefore, that authoritarian leadership "is probably the worst [thing] that a leader would ever inflict upon a group of people."

Her decision for a participative style was also born out of a sense of dual respect: a respect of people and for knowledge. The following segment from the transcript illustrates these beliefs as well as her clear self-assuredness.

> I recognize that there is a very great deal of power in a position but it is not half as good, not half as lasting, as the power of knowledge and if you rationally decide and have a group decision —then it works, because people are committed to it. I don't think there is any question about that. I am quite sure I was a good dean. I think I was a democratic dean and our faculty meetings had people bouncing up all the time to have their ideas presented —it got a little hot sometimes, but that was good.

Rozella used these same principles as she conceived the collaboration model or the experiment in nursing, as it was also known. She was interested in developing a model in which the power of influence was exerted, rather than the power of autocracy. As Rozella said, the collaboration model was "a new approach to relating two interdependent institutions so that neither lost its autonomy and the objectives of both would be fulfilled."

This experiment in nursing was, literally, an experiment, designed to

> envision a better future and then take action to create it . . . an experiment which we predicted would facilitate the improvement of nursing care and education and the advancement of nursing knowledge. The experiment involved the creation of a new relationship between the university's school of nursing and the university hospitals. It required substantial change in the methods of operating in the two institutions. (Schlotfeldt & MacPhail, 1969a, p. 1018)

This collaboration model, was born out of her experiences at Iowa and Wayne. At Iowa, there was close involvement between practice and education with resultant good nursing practice. However, nursing instructors were also nursing supervisors who had dual appointments or "200 percent" commitments. At Wayne, nursing practice had suffered because of the complete separation of the School of Nursing from the responsibility for the clinical sites. Seeing both ends of this continuum, Rozella resolved, "It's neither right to have complete separation of education from service, not is it right to have them to be one in the same. I had to find a way to do it." At Frances Payne Bolton School of Nursing, therefore, she established a model in which the heads of clinical departments were the heads in both practice and education with 50/50 appointments in each institution. The directors were the policy makers, expected to return to their departments and share information and responsibility, thus decentralizing authority. The nursing organization in the hospital was modeled after the medical staff organization. "I'm a great admirer of medicine," says Rozella in discussing her decision, "it has everything I want . . . . If we're going to emulate any group, why not the MDs?" Also reasoning that "if you want to change a role, you change a title and get new expectations around it," the nurses were given different titles. More rigorous educational requirements were also established for nurses. The roles and responsibilities were being defined as they were being practiced, with constant designing, defining, and reevaluation. The continuing commitment throughout was Rozella's determination to think of a new way to relate the faculty of the School of Nursing to the practice setting. The faculty, she argued, "deprived not only themselves but also their students" by distancing from practice, because "the questions were not forthcoming."

(I will not discuss her paradigm on the nature of nursing other than to say that she believes in collaborative, collegial, professional practice among those in the various health care disciplines, and she believes that nursing practice must be grounded in knowledge born of research.)

The third contribution Rozella counts as significant is her early work on conceptualizing the Nursing Doctorate (ND). As she states, "We already have programs that recognize that nursing is a complex profession and that we should have first professional degrees that are based upon liberalizing education and a strong scientific, humanistic base." Thus, holding strong beliefs in the value of a liberalizing education, and finding herself unsatisfied with the amount of knowledge that students of nursing had, Rozella "began cooking in my head about the ND."

It was an educational model designed to give students a solid foundation in nursing's knowledge base prior to caring for patients: shifting the emphasis from learning how to *do* to learning how to *know*. As Rozella says, "Nothing like knowledge!"

The pervasiveness of the androcentric society is clearly seen influencing her life. The apparent contradictions, equivocations, deference, and qualifications in judgments about self or others reflective of women's oppression *is* also evidenced in her life. However, Rozella Schlotfeldt is a woman who has made acclaimed contributions to nursing against great odds imposed by living and practicing her profession in an oppressive society. She was able to do this because of the networks of love and support from other women and her own personal persistence to overcome adversity.

REFERENCES

Ashley, J. A. (1980). Power in structured misogyny: Implications for the politics of care. *Advances in Nursing Science, 23*(2), 3–21.

Atkinson, T. G. (1978). Radical feminism. In M. B. Mahowald (Ed.) (1983). *Philosophy of woman: An anthology of classic and current concepts* (2nd ed.). Indianapolis: Hackett Publishing Co.

Bernard, J. (1985). The marital bond vis-a-vis the male bond and the female bond. *AFTA Newsletter, 19*, 15–22.

Bowen, M. (1978). *Family therapy in clinical practice.* New York: Jason Aronson, Inc.

Callaway, H. (1981). Women's perspectives: Research as re-vision. In P. Reason & J. Rowan. *Human inquiry: A sourcebook of new paradigm research* (pp. 457–471). New York: John Wiley & Sons.

Chinn, P. (1982). What's in our name??? *Cassandra: Radical Feminist Nurses Newsletter, 1*(1), 3–5.

Chinn, P. & Wheeler, C. E. (1985). Feminism and nursing: Can nursing afford to remain aloof from the women's movement? *Nursing Outlook, 33*(2), 74–77.

Christy, T. (1971). Equal rights for women: Voices from the past. *American Journal of Nursing, 71*(2), 288–293.

Cleland, V. (1971). Sex discrimination: Nursing's most pervasive problem. *American Journal of Nursing, 71*(8), 1542–1547.

Christ, C. P., & Plaskow, J. (Eds.) (1979). *Womanspirit rising: A feminist reader in religion.* New York: Harper & Row.

Cook, B. W. (1977). Female support networks and political activism: Lillian Wald, Crystal Eastman, Emma Goldman. *Chrysalis, 3*, 43–61.

Daly, M. (1978). *Gyn/ecology: The metaethics of radical feminism.* Boston: Beacon Press.

Friedan, B. (1970). Our revolution is unique. In M. B. Mahowald (Ed.). (1983). *Philosophy of woman: An anthology of classic and current concepts* (2nd ed.). Indianapolis: Hackett Publishing Co.

Frye, M. (1983). *The politics of reality: Essays in feminist theory.* Trumansburg, NY: The Crossing Press.

Janeway, E. (1971). *Man's world, woman's place: A study in social mythology.* New York: William Morrow and Company, Inc.

Kolbenschlag, M. (1979). *Kiss Sleeping Beauty Good-bye.* New York: Bantam Books.

Mahowald, M. B. (Ed.). (1983). *Philosophy of woman: An anthology of classic and current concepts* (2nd ed.). Indianapolis: Hackett Publishing Co.

Palmer, I. S. (1986). Research on nursing's heritage. In H. H. Werley & J. J. Fitzpatrick (Eds.), *Annual review of nursing research, 4,* New York: Springer.

Radford Ruether, R. (1983). *Sexism and God-talk: Toward a feminist theology.* Boston: The Beacon Press.

Raymand, J. (1982). A geneology of female friendship. *Trivia: A Journal of Ideas, 1*(1), 11.

Russell, L. M. (Ed.). (1976). *The liberating word: A guide to nonsexist interpretation of the Bible.* Philadelphia: The Westminister Press.

Schlotfeldt, R. M. & MacPhail, J. (1969a). Experiment in nursing: Characteristics and rationale, *American Journal of Nursing, 69*(5), 1018–1023.

Schussler Fiorenza, E. (1983). *In memory of her: A feminist theological reconstruction of Christian origins.* New York: Crossroad.

Steinem, G. (1983). *Outrageous acts and everyday rebellions.* New York: Holt, Rinehart and Winston.

Wilson-Kastner, P. (1983). *Faith, feminism & the Christ.* Philadelphia: Fortress Press.

Wood, J. T. (1982). *Human communication: A symbolic interactionist perspective.* New York: Holt, Rinehart and Winston.

6

The Context of Feminism and Nursing in 19th-Century Victorian England

Marylouise Welch

Writing in *Hidden From History*, Sheila Rowbotham (1976) makes the case for women examining their past. The history of women has been silent and neglectful of the women's voice. "It is evident that the rediscovery of our history is an essential aspect of the creation of a feminist critique of male culture" (p. xvii). This paper then examines the life of Florence Nightingale in the culture of mid-19th-century Victorian England and explores how her own personal experiences coupled with the status of women and the events of the times shaped her development as well as the emergence of the profession of nursing.

Nightingale was born in 1820 to an upper middle-class English family residing in Florence, Italy. When not on the continent the family spent their time between their country homes Lea Hurst and Embley and rented apartments in London for the "season." At the time of Florence's birth, England was predominantly a two-class society. The complacent and self-satisfied upper class lived with contentment and indifference while the lower classes were oppressed paupers plagued by illness and early death.

During her formative years, Florence always identified more with her father than her mother. He was a Unitarian and an ardent supporter of Jeremy

Bentham and social liberalism. Unitarians were striving to create a more perfect world focusing on justice, and had a long tradition of support for the
emancipation of women. Nightingale's education was influenced and directed
by her father. While Florence was young, her father recognized her keen
mind and sought to develop it with her. He hired tutors to provide for her a
classical education including Latin and Greek and 18th-century philosophy.
He was a man of ideas and brought many intellectuals to the home on week-
ends where dinner conversation included lively sharing and debating of current social and political issues.

Florence's relationship with her mother was characterized by bitter conflict and a battle of will over the proper role for a lady in Victorian society.
Both her mother and her sister fought against and obstructed Florence in the
realization of her desires for many years. Several biographers have suggested
that the lack of support and loneliness that Florence felt contributed to her
disdain for women in her later life.

As she continued to feel more isolated from the daily routines of her family,
Florence turned to religion and spirituality for comfort. She was moved by the
writings of early mystics of the Catholic church like Teresa of Avila and
considered converting to Catholicism. In 1837, she had a vision in which God
spoke with her and convinced her that her life should be in service to Him.
She wrote in her diary, "I desire for a considerable time only to lead a life of
obscurity and toil for the purpose of allowing whatever I may have received
of God to ripen; and turning it some day to the glory of his name" (in Cook,
1913). This theme was woven into the context of the rest of her life.

For the next few years while in her early twenties Florence was a confused,
disheartened young woman. She was aware of her own intellectual gifts but
she was also tormented by the clash between her desire to marry and fulfill
her mother's expectations and her knowledge that this role would ultimately
leave her dissatisfied. She participated with her mother in what she sarcasti-
cally named "poor peopling," doing token gestures for the poor and the sick
but never making a commitment or getting involved. In 1844, she had a significant conversation with Dr. Samuel Howe while he was visiting with his
wife Julia Ward Howe at Embley. This encounter solidified her desire to
devote her energy and intelligence to the care of the sick.

Her personal education had been influenced by her tutored study of the
classics and the writings of Newton, Locke, Condorcet, Compte, and her
contemporaries, Mill and Jowett. These intellectuals, though approaching the
question from different perspectives, were examining the notion that human
existence was as subject to natural laws as other components of the universe
and that these laws might be discovered through rigorous application of scientific principles. Concurrently, they also investigated the relationships of man,

nature, and the state. Questions about the existence of God and the role of religion in people's lives arose and this issue became a lively debate in early 19th-century intellectual circles.

As Nightingale tried to clarify her own beliefs, she wrote a three-volume treatise entitled *Suggestions for Thought for Seekers After Truth Among the Artisans of England*. There were very few copies of this work printed and it was not until the 20th century that historians were able to examine it. A true discussion of this document is for another time but there are several faiths and doubts that she expresses in this work that remain with her throughout her life.

In this work, she presented an eclectic personal philosophy that examined these broad notions and what she believed about them. Margaret Newton (1949) summarizes Nightingale's philosophic inquiry as follows: (1) She held ardent faith in God as First Causee, Creator, and Law giver, and that God's laws were immutable but that people were capable of learning and growing and improving through knowledge of these Laws. (2) Knowledge was gained through experience and from the senses, and she remained forever the observer, reflector, empiricist. It is important to note that during her life Pasteur, Lister, Darwin, and Marx were all making discoveries and writing about them. (3) Life was dynamic, it was good and inevitable that all things were subject to change. If people worked hard and gained enough knowledge, then much of the world's ignorance and suffering would be alleviated. This tenet was a very common 19th-century belief about how simple it could be to improve the human condition.

Finally, of most significance to this discussion, there is in the appendix a work entitled *Cassandra* in which Nightingale describes her despair that society makes no commitment to the development of women's gifts and talents. The following quotations were taken from a section of *Cassandra* subtitled "The Household Prisoner."

> *Why have women passion, intellect and moral activity—these three—and a place in society where none of these three can be exercised?*

> *Mrs. A. has the imagination of the poetry of Murillo . . . why is she not a Murillo? . . . If she has a knife and fork in her hands for three hours of the day, she cannot have a pencil and a brush.*

Nightingale was aware that the century was on the brink of new knowledge and exciting discoveries from which women would be excluded. During this period she states that she is committed to freeing women of the burden of the family by bringing to their lives the direction of the mystical God.

Thus, here is a woman who sought to develop her intellectual and practical skills and who turned to nursing for fulfillment. In 1851, despite tremendous opposition from her family, Nightingale served for a short time in Kaiserworth, Germany, with Pastor Fliedner who had established a 100-bed hospital and community service agency for the sick and the poor. She stayed there for three months and actually attended a course at the Kaiserworth Institute for the Training of Deaconesses. Finally, in 1853, she became the Superintendent of the Establishment for Gentlewomen During Illness. Here she learned to maneuver and manipulate and gained her first insights into her talents as an administrator (Smith, 1982).

Nightingale was serving at this post when she was asked by Sidney Herbert, the Secretary of War, to lead a group of nurses to the Crimea. She left for the Crimea as the Superintendent of a group of 40 nurses some of whom were lay people and most were Sisters of Charity.

At 33, as she embarks on the most significant adventure in her life, she can be compared with some other lesser known Victorian women leaders. Harriet Martineau, who was a personal friend, never married, and helped foster changes in the opportunities for and attitudes toward the work and education of unmarried women. Josephine Butler exposed the poverty as well as the male sexual desires that gave rise to prostitution. She brought attention to the fact that prostitutes were victims of an insensitive society. Elizabeth Fry read to inmates at Newgate prison and tried to pioneer reform for women prisoners. Otavia Hill founded the National Trust, the English Conservancy, and the profession of social work.

All these women came from privileged educated backgrounds. Boyd (1982) describes their efforts as an attempt to reform society and to meet the needs of Great Britain in the light of the ideal Christian community. Their efforts were from within the then current system for reform and for a role for women. Recently, they have been ignored by leading feminists because they evolved from the Christian ethic, although through their efforts the status and education of all women were improved. For them the demand of service to God and to society as a whole took precedence over the rights of women.

Thus, as Nightingale departed for the Crimea, she was also a Christian feminist serving God by serving a group in need, but not, at the same time, committed to the cause of releasing women from male dominance and oppression. This was espoused by an alternate feminist movement in England exemplified by the work of Emmeline Pankhurst and Barbara Smith and dedicated to the emancipation of women and women's right to vote (Herstein, 1985). These feminists rebelled against the then current situation and believed that the world should change so that women and men were equal in the eyes of the law as well as equal in the home. As I will discuss later, when Nightingale returned from the Crimea both types of feminists called upon her for support.

The account of Nightingale's accomplishments at Scutari is well known. She arrived to find chaos, no supplies, and a mortality rate among the wounded of 47 percent, which far exceeded the mortality rate in battle. Within six months of her arrival, the mortality rate for the wounded had shrunk to 2.2 percent (Cohen, 1984). She had many struggles with men in command of the army and medical care, and also with many of the women who were a part of her original group of 40 nurses as well as with another group of nurses who arrived soon after she did. She became an authoritarian and controlling administrator, and she came to view this approach as the only method for righting a chaotic system in order to improve the health of the soldiers (Smith, 1982).

Nightingale's experience in the Crimea solidified many of her early views. She was ultimately practical. She viewed women as doers and she believed the knowledge in which she could place the most confidence was that which she had gained by experience. She remained forever to trust her own personal experiences over any new scientific data including the revelations by Lister and Pasteur regarding germ theory.

Nightingale returned in poor health and ever more skeptical of women. She wrote to her dear friend Mary Clarke Mohl that women with whom she had worked in the Crimea had learned nothing of permanent value and described them as being incompetent and incapable of original thought (Woodham-Smith, 1951). She withdrew immediately from the spotlight, often never leaving her bedroom for weeks at a time (Cook, 1913). She developed the "Nightingale Cabinet" comprised solely of men willing to help her further her work and her goals. She did the research, developed the statistics and comparative data, and wrote the white papers which her "cabinet" then took to the appropriate boards to ensure the passage of her recommendations (Cohen, 1984). Everything she undertook was intended to improve the life of the soldiers and the citizens of the Empire. She had been thunderstruck by the neglect and unnecessary deaths and conditions at Scutari and she returned committed forever to serve the soldiers of the Empire. The following are two quotations that she entered in her diary concerning the situation there:

Oh, my poor men, I am a bad mother to come home and leave you to your Crimean graves.
I stand at the altar of the murdered men and while I live I fight their cause.

Mildred E. Newton (1949) summarizes her accomplishments through the period 1856 to 1880 as follows: (1) improved and reformed laws affecting health and the poor, (2) reformed hospitals and workhouses, (3) organized an army medical school, (4) improved health for British subjects at home and in the colonies, and (5) established nursing as a profession.

Nightingale's ardent concern for women so evident in *Cassandra* is no longer present. The demands of service to God and the British people took precedence over the rights of women. She did not identify with people who were concerned with the suffrage movement and oppression by men. She herself was not oppressed, when, with the stroke of a pen, she could bring the Prime Minister to her bedroom. She no longer personally felt powerless. Furthermore, her family and Crimean experiences had taught her to trust men not women. She remained as removed from the cause of feminism as she did from society at large. Nevertheless, during these years, she was called on to support a feminist perspective from several divergent groups.

For example, Nightingale chose not to work with Elizabeth Blackwell, the first woman physician, who wished to establish a free-standing woman's hospital with training school for nurses and women physicians. Blackwell believed that the school would attract upper class well-educated women who would need very minimal education to become nurses. Then, after having achieved this first phase of training, these women would move out of nursing into medical education that would be academic and rigorous.

Nightingale disagreed with the Blackwell plan on several counts. First, she perceived it would be doomed by the powerful medical establishment which would muster political support in opposition. She also disagreed with the outlined educational process. She saw an elitism in this plan that was not her intent. She wrote her response to Blackwell in a letter stating, "you wish to educate a few highly cultivated ones . . . I wish to diffuse as much knowledge as possible (in Monteiro, 1984)." If she relinquished the 60,000 pounds raised for nursing by the soldiers of the Crimea to this scheme, she would be forced to share authority and control. She had become too distrustful to ever put her self in the position of sharing power. Finally, Nightingale was not the same type of feminist that Blackwell was. She believed women should develop their talents in arenas in which they had special abilities and not just with the motive to do something "merely because men do it." She was primarily an individualist encouraging people to develop their own unique gifts without consideration of gender. She summarizes this view at the end of *Notes on Nursing* (1859) in a Postscript: "I would earnestly ask my sisters of . . . the jargon, namely about the rights of women, which urges women to do all that men do, including the medical and other professions, merely because men do it, and without regard to whether this is the best that women can do." Nightingale also criticized women who entered the field of medicine and adapted themselves to a male model rather than using their unique qualities to bring about improvement in health care.

In 1867, Nightingale offers a second example of her lost interest in the cause of women's rights. When her old friend John Stuart Mill sought her assistance in his campaign for women's suffrage, she was willing to sign the petition but not to make it her cause. She was involved in many other issues that took precedence. In fact, in 1858 she wrote to Harriet Martineau, "I am brutally indifferent to the wrongs of my sex" (Cook, 1913).

At this point Mill had written *The Subjection of Women* (1870) which was his logical argument for the equality of women. He approached the women's issue from both the utilitarian perspective, which analyzed the position of women in society, and from the liberal perspective, which emphasised women's potential for growth and learning (Randall, 1984). However, no where did Mill exhibit an understanding of the situation of the women of the lower classes. For example, he states that women should not have to contribute to the finances of the family and yet, for most women, this was not a social reality. When all the liberal reformers including Mill voted for the Mining Act that removed women from the mines, they did not recognize that these women now had no other source of employment. Often, the liberals operated from an academic rather than a perspective based in the economic reality of oppression. For all of Nightingale's faults, it was she who was grounded in the economic and social reality of women. And nursing became for her the one occupation in which women could gain education and respectability as well as an income, however meager.

Finally, I perceive Nightingale's feminism as an extention of the Victorian concept of mother. When thinking of the derivation of the word *nursing* and its roots in the maternal caring instinct, what better metaphor from which to view Nightingale than as the mother of humankind. Her achievements in nursing, hospital reform, and improvement in the status of women were secondary accomplishments all leading to the goal of improving the life of the British citizen.

In *Cassandra*, written in her youth, she criticized parents for not nurturing and enabling their children, but instead selfishly requiring their children to live as they lived. Her ideal parent develops self-confidence in children that empowers them to move out into the world and lead independent lives serving God. When she returned from the Crimea, she had been very much the nurturing caring mother of the soldier, rather similar to Queen Victoria, the ultimate mother to the Empire and a woman with whom she shared both affection and similar experiences.

While in the Crimea, Nightingale received correspondence from the Queen encouraging her in her endeavor and allowing Nightingale to use the Queen's influence when it was necessary to achieve her goals (Cook, 1913). Upon her return, she was received by the Queen and the Prince Consort at Balmoral. Neither of these women wished to become feminists, in fact each saw herself always working for and through men (Auerback, 1982). They were each working with a cabinet of men on whom they relied to accomplish their goals. They were both viewed by the public as women alone and in command and their role as mother to the soldier and citizen of the Empire became a myth and a legacy of the Victorian Era. Both women used and enjoyed power and through their maternal positions were able to control the man as well as the boy.

Nightingale's nursing administration power developed because of her maternal caring response to the overwhelming loss of life that she witnessed at Scutari. From that experience she had come to accept the responsibility as mother to the family of England, to be care provider to the world at large, and to work for social reform. To do the Lord's work was to extend the maternal metaphor by promoting health and by caring for and healing the dying and the sick.

Modern nursing's birth stems from this conservative feminist position with its roots in Christian idealism and its emphasis on women's talents for doing rather than thinking. However, this birthright has been an onerous burden for women and for the profession of nursing. As Nightingale experienced life she felt women's "lack of sympathy" (in Cook, 1913) and came to believe that it was only in men that she could put her trust. She left the profession dominated by men and by medicine. She never seemed to understand that the education and freedom she had attained for herself would be necessary for all women in all professions.

REFERENCES

Auerback, N. (1982). *Woman and the demon: The life of a Victorian myth.* Cambridge: Harvard University Press.

Boyd, N. (1982). *Three Victorian women who changed their world.* New York: Oxford University Press.

Cohen, B. (1984). Florence Nightingale. *Scientific American, 250*(3), 128–137.

Cook, E. (1913). *The life of Florence Nightingale.* London: MacMillan.

Herstein, S. R. (1985). *Mid-Victorian feminist. Barbara Leigh Smith Bodichon.* New Haven: Yale University Press.

Mill, J. S. (1870). *The subjection of women.* New York: D. Appleton.

Monteiro, L. A. (1984). On separate roads: Florence Nightingale and Elizabeth Blackwell. *Signs: Journal of Women in Culture and Society, 9*(31).

Newton, M. E. (1949). *Florence Nightingale's philosophy of life and education.* Unpublished doctoral dissertation. Stanford, CA: Stanford University.

Nightingale, F. (1859). *Notes on nursing.* London: Harrison & Sons.

Nightingale, F. (1859). *Notes on hospitals.* London: Harrison & Sons.

Nightingale, F. (1860). *Suggestions for thought to searchers after truths among the artizans of England.* London: Eyre & Spottiswoode.

Nightingale, F. (1860). *Suggestions for thought to searchers after religious truths, Vol. II and Vol. III.* London: Eyre & Spottiswoode.

Nightingale, F. (1873). A note of interrogation. *Fraser's Magazine (New Series),* 7(5), 567–577.

Nightingale, F. (1873). A sub-note of interrogation: What will our religion be in 1999? *Fraser's Magazine (New Series),* 8(7), 25–36.

Nightingale, F. (1882). Training of nurses. In R. Quain (Ed.), *A dictionary of medicine* (pp. 1038–1043). London: Longman's Green Company.

Palmer, I. (1976). Florence Nightingale and the Salisbury incident. *Nursing Research, 25,* 370–377.

Palmer, I. (1977). Florence Nightingale: Reformer, reactionary, researcher. *Nursing Research, 26,* 84–89.

Palmer, I. (1981). Florence Nightingale and the international origins of modern nursing. *Image, 13*(2), 28–31.

Palmer, I. (1983). Nightingale revisited. *Nursing Outlook, 31,* 229–233.

Randall, J. (1984). *The origins of modern feminism: Women in Britain, France and the United States, 1780–1860.* New York: Schocken Books.

Reimer, E., & Fout, J. (Eds.). (1980). *European women.* New York: Schocken Books.

Rowbotham, S. (1976). *Hidden from history: Rediscovering women in history from the 17th century to the present.* New York: Vintage Books.

Smith, F. B. (1982). *Florence Nightingale: Reputation and power.* London: Croom Helm.

Strachey, L. (1920). *Emminent Victorians.* New York: Garden City Publishing Company.

Woodham-Smith, C. (1951). *Florence Nightingale.* New York: McGraw-Hill.

This paper, an expanded version of the article, "Florence Nightingale—The Social Construction of a Victorian Feminist," originally published in *Western Journal of Nursing Research,* Vol. 12, No. 3, pp. 404–407, is reprinted here with permission of © Sage Publications, Inc.

7

The Feminist Movement and the Science and Profession of Nursing: Analogies and Paradoxes

Patricia S. Yaros

INTRODUCTION

To state that social change is glacial is to state a truism without any insight. To gain insight into the extraordinarily slow changes in the world for women, one must examine the forces which have circumscribed women's situations in this world. Nursing, as a profession and a science, has selectively deflected and absorbed the enforced subordination, limited options, and social powerlessness of women as a whole. In this paper, I will present analogies and paradoxes in both the development of the feminist movement and in the development of nursing as a science and a profession. Such an examination should yield implications and direction for both feminism and nursing.

Margaret Forster (1984) has observed that there really has not been a women's movement that has steadily progressed through the decades. Rather, women have episodically organized for the achievement of a particular goal and then experienced some dissolution of their "movement" (whether the goal was realized or not). As a result, "Feminism, because of this, is not like a political belief. You cannot join the feminist party, for example . . ." (p. 1). Although there are many women's organizations you can join, the world is not structured so that you can say, "I am a feminist" in the same way you can say, "I am a Republican."

As it was in the 19th century, it is still necessary to ask a woman if she is a feminist. Why have not the enormous rank and file of women been attracted to the concepts of feminism? Likewise, why have not the vast majority of nurses sought recognition and autonomy in the professional arena? Timidity and turmoil from Nightingale's time to now describes the context of nursing as an underpaid workforce. Nurses, as the largest single group of health care providers, potentially command great political power. Yet such power has not been realized. The science in which nurses could potentially embed their practice has not been translatable to bedside care.

BACKGROUND CONCEPTS

Critical concepts that expand our understanding of the analogies and para-doxes of feminism and nursing include: power and powerlessness, domination and subordination, and restrictions and options. The impact of these concepts has been significant to the life experiences of women and of women as nurses. The challenge to nurses and to women is to understand this impact without being confined to the abstract. To examine what has been real and to learn from such examination can become a force of empowerment for women and nurses in the future.

When exposing the philosophical roots of power, domination, and restric-tions, a traditional patriarchal and hierarchical dualism becomes evident. In this hierarchy, the first half of the dualism sees itself as fundamentally better than the second. This is certainly true in the case of sexual dualism, one sex as better than the other; in the case of class, one class as better than others; or in cultures, one race or species as better than another (Griscom, 1985). "Thus the superior half is entitled to more power than the inferior—power over, needless to say, not power for" (p. 89). Inferior groups can then be objectified, used, and exploited as resources.

Furthermore, power means that when those with power say, "This is the way it is," then that is the way it is believed to be. The powerful have a unique credibility carried beyond a rightful and legitimate knowledge base. The world adapts itself to what the powerful want to see as true. Actually, that is not always so, but if it appears to be, it is because power constructs the appearance of reality by silencing the voices of the powerless, by excluding them from access to authoritative discourse. In contrast, the powerless do not have the same credibility as the powerful. When the powerless say, "This is the way it is," it is rarely taken as being that way in fact.

In a woman's world, this also means that gender structures a system of social hierarchy, a political arena of male dominance and female subordination, and an insidious socialization where women come to believe that they have a survival stake in the system that suppresses them. In the nurses's world, the analogy can be made that the medical monopoly on health care has enforced a subordination of nurses, exploited their ideas and talents, and given nurses no-win options in dealing with the existing health care enterprise.

HISTORICAL ANALOGIES AND PARADOXES IN FEMINISM AND NURSING

From the grassroots of feminism to the foundations of nursing, there has been shared history and shared ideas. Although at one time in her life Florence Nightingale claimed she was not a feminist, the impact of her work on both nursing and feminism was monumental. There was, according to Nightingale, an intimate lived relationship between the two. At some time in each woman's life it would be necessary to care for the personal health of another. As such, every woman lived nursing for a shorter or greater length of time and intensity of involvement. Nightingale then marveled at what a valuable product would result if all women's total nursing experiences could be translated to help one *think* how to nurse (Nightingale, 1969, p. 4).

Although the Nightingale thesis of woman and nurse were valuable early conceptualizations of what nursing was, there were troublesome underpinnings to that thesis that even she wanted to avoid. At that time, the new woman could achieve some prestige for doing what she was already doing and what was considered natural for her to do. This followed the general (male) belief that a woman's ability to think was strongly linked to her body and her sexuality, and that her brain was physiologically different (inferior) to the male brain. All of this served to restrict women's options and channel them to well-controlled (male-controlled) arenas. When women gave voice to the frustrations such false limitations imposed, some social concern was expressed. However, this concern avoided the cause of women's frustrations preferring to consider what was wrong with women and also indirectly what was problematic about their aspirations (Church & Poirier, 1986). Even quite recently have I heard a male physician say "what's the matter with you nurses, what do you want to do, get rid of physicians?"

In *Notes on Nursing* (1859/1969), Nightingale strongly cautioned that women should not listen to exhortations to not choose a certain kind of work because it was unseemly for a woman, or to do any work just because a man could do it. She strongly urged women to do well whatever suited them best to do. Perhaps we are just now getting to the point that young women are truly investing their energies in any profession that they wish, not only the traditional women's professions. At the same time, it's also getting far rarer to see a woman spotlighted for her uniqueness in a traditional men's occupation.

A tangential side to applauding women who can succeed in any occupation is to examine the woman who "strives to lose her female identity, or to go beyond it, to be regarded *as a person* in a world that grants the status of persons only to men" (Raymond, 1985). Such women frequently view themselves free from the "world of traditional women as well as from the world of feminist women" (p. 170). They take pains to proclaim that they have moved beyond feminism. The irony of this disidentification is that these women engage in quite extraordinary activities that *are* feminist in the sense that these endeavors require unconventional capabilities, courage, determination, and persistence. We see these women as scientists, truck drivers, telephone repair people, deans of schools of nursing, and directors of nursing service who are often more astute and humane than men in the same fields, but, when asked, would deny woman-identification.

As a corollary, how many of us, when asked what we do, answer, I am a nurse (our fundamental identification). If we are in a college of nursing, do we only answer, "I teach at the university," or if in a hospital, "I work at the hospital." What does this tell us about a denial of our identity? What does this tell us about our quest for status? What does this tell us about how pervasive the subordination of women as nurses is.

In nursing's history, there are a number of women who went beyond the subordination and limitations imposed by society. Margaret Sanger comes to mind immediately. In the early 1900s, Sanger "challenged political and social institutions head-on and won" (Ruffing-Rahal, 1986). At the time, any information on birth control, other than for disease prevention, was strictly illegal and what contraception was available was male-controlled. Then, at the deathbed of one of her patients, Sanger renounced nursing within the medical system to tend to the wider social and ethical problem of women's lack of control over their own bodies. Is that an answer for nursing—to completely renounce our identity with the title "nurse" as some would suggest? What irony, that to be fully an independent thinking woman is seen as unwomanly, and perhaps to fully realize the capabilities of being a nurse, we may not be called "nurse."

Peggy Chinn (1988) recently remarked that:

> As nurses we are particularly vulnerable to an unrelenting sense of disparity between what we know and what we do. We know we

would be stronger as a profession if we were unified with each other and with other health care providers, but we are not unified. We know we would be able to provide a high quality of care if we were free to practice nursing as we envision it to be, but we do not and cannot practice in these ways. We know we would better serve society if we focused our practice on health and developed greater knowledge about health, but we practice in an illness care system, and not a health care system. (p. vii)

Does it not follow that also as women we know we would have greater power to shape a more peaceful world if we had unity? Could we not as women better serve society, our families, ourselves, if we focused on the issues which we know will help the survival of our world even as we live in a world often violent, with sometimes cruel and senseless endings to life.

Encouraging signs include new "women's movements." At this time, we have Mothers Against Drunk Driving—a force changing legislation, judges, legislators, and death statistics. But also in the last two decades we've seen the emergence of battered women's shelters, rape crisis centers, women's health clinics, and women's studies programs. A warning must be sounded that some of these have been temporary or unsuccessful because they follow the episodic nature of feminists' ventures where there is a communion of resistance and nothing more. This should tell us again that unity for broader purposes will enhance survival of feminist initiatives.

MODERN FEMINISM AND NURSING'S ANALOGIES AND PARADOXES

Where do we stand in the new movements in nursing? The science and study of nursing has been profoundly influenced by the status as a women's profession subordinate to other "experts." The socialization of women as inferior men still touches aspects of our science and our practice. The borrowing of theories with little regard for application to nursing's concerns could be said to be another example of shame for our own identity. Nursing-identified models such as Rogers' are held in suspicion and ridiculed for their language and the abstractness.

Nor would this be the first time you have heard that nursing has been coopted by the medical model. Historically, physician domination in the health field has resulted in the "medicalization of life," where the physician, by virtue of transforming even social and ethical problems into pieces of the medical pie, becomes the resident expert on a wide area of human life (Figlio, 1977). Remember that power has this credible voice. The medical model has so excluded other voices that you may scarcely find a member of the public who does not believe that medicine does have all the answers.

Allan and Hall (1988) have debunked the myth of the medical model in a recent paper, where they link the Cartesian foundations of medical science to a dehumanizing and technological view of human life which pervades our society. They illustrate how the medical model promotes the concept of disease as being separate from the person, excludes the human from the environment, and attempts to reduce all life phenomena to singular causations. As women and as nurses, this is antagonistic and contradictory to our personal and professional life experiences. Our science base has caught up with these beliefs and has promise of validating a view of the contextual nature of the human experience, including all experiences of health and illness, through new research methodologies unique to nursing. We also have the beginnings of the feminist perspective within nursing's theory-building research.

We will shed the paradoxes of our history as women and as nurses when we unify for common proactive not reactive purposes, providing creative and appropriate interchanges that promote common goals. A woman's model, the feminist model, could better serve to unify and not divide—the feminist model of collaboration, not competition, and of sharing, not hoarding. We have many caring women in nursing with many contributions—I'm speaking of the housekeepers who converse with hospitalized patients, the nursing scientists who search for valid nursing measures, the emergency room and intensive care nurses who make split-second life-saving decisions, and the public health and clinic nurses who care for families and communities. What a vision of the future, with women and nurses in the caring professions working together in a feminist model.

Maggie Kuhn, one of the prime movers of the Gray Panthers, spoke at this year's American Nurses' Association convention, urging nurses to be the ethical advocates in shaping a new health care system for all Americans. She's a woman who proudly proclaims, "I am an old woman, not a senior citizen." She shared with us what she wanted her tombstone to read: "Here lies Maggie Kuhn, above her stands the only stone she left unturned." Wouldn't we all, as feminists and as nurses, like to be able to say that?

REFERENCES

Ashley, J. A. (1975). Nurses and early feminism. *American Journal of Nursing,* 75, 1465–1467.

Chinn, P. (1988). Knowing and doing. *Advances in Nursing Science, 10*(3), vii–viii.

Church, O. M., & Poirier, S. (1986). From patient to consumer; from apprentice to professional practitioner. *Nursing Clinics of North America, 21*(1), 99–109.

Deckard, B. S. (1979). *The women's movement: Political, socioeconomic, and psychological issues,* (2nd ed.). New York: Harper & Row.

Figlio, K. (1977). The historiography of scientific medicine: An invitation to the human sciences. *Comparative Studies in Social History, 19,* 262–286.

Forster, M. (1984). *Significant sisters.* New York: Oxford University Press.

Griscom, J. L. (1985). On healing the nature/history split in feminist thought. In B. H. Andolsen, C. E. Gudorf, & M. D. Pellauer (Eds.), *Women's consciousness, women's conscience: A reader in feminist ethics* (pp. 85–98). Minneapolis: Winston Press.

MacKinnon, C. A. (1987). *Feminism unmodified: Discourses on life and law.* Cambridge: Harvard University Press.

Nightingale, F. (1969). *Notes on nursing: What it is, and what it is not.* New York: Dover Publications. (Original work published 1859).

O'Brien, P. (1987). "All a woman's life can bring": The domestic roots of nursing in Philadelphia, 1830–1885. *Nursing Research, 36*(1), 12–17.

Parsons, M. (1986). The profession in a class by itself. *Nursing Outlook, 34*(6), 270–275.

Raymond, J. (1985). Female friendship and feminist ethics. In B. H. Andolsen, C. E. Gudorf, & M. D. Pellauer (Eds.), *Women's consciousness, women's conscience: A reader in feminist ethics* (pp. 161–174). Minneapolis: Winston Press.

Ruffing-Rahal, M. (1986). Margaret Sanger: Nurse and feminist. *Nursing Outlook, 34*(5), 246–249.

Wheeler, C. E. (1985). The American journal of nursing and the socialization of a profession, 1900–1920. *Advances in Nursing Science, 7*(2), 20–34.

8

Professional Nurse Caring: A Conceptual Model for Nursing

Carol Green-Hernandez

CARING: A FEMININE CONSTRUCT

The *what* of caring is a subject of much debate among nursing as well as feminist scholars. Leininger (1977), Watson (1979), and Gaut (1979) all state that caring is nursing's essence. Gilligan (1982) asserts that care is the basis for binding individuals together in interpersonal connection. When viewed as a commitment to caring, such connection provides a basis for nurturance. Noddings (1984) believes that caring as nurturance is a feminine capability. Her view grounds a moral vision of caring which is distinctly feminist, for caring is seen as deriving from the nurturance inherent in connected relationship rather than the less-connected, the focus of traditional androgeny. This author would add these feminist views to the statement that caring is nursing's essence (Leininger, 1977; Watson, 1979; Gaut, 1979). That is, the nurse's ability to practice professional caring derives from a feminine-connectedness with both client(s) and colleagues.

DEVELOPMENT AND SUBSEQUENT
VALIDATION OF THE MODEL

The foregoing contention provides the basis for a proposed conceptual model for nursing. This model emerged from a two-fold analytic approach which supported its conceptualization. First, a far-ranging literature review of theologic, philosophic, behavioral science (psychology and sociology), medical, and nursing domains provided the content for a philosophic, inductive "dwelling with" the concept of caring as it related to humankind and, specifically, nursing. Second, the conceptualization of caring that emerged from this process provided the organizing framework for several qualitative investigations of the lived experience of caring in nurses (Hernandez, 1985, 1987, 1988a, 1989; Ingle, 1987b, 1988; Burns, under investigation). Results from these studies suggest that caring is a concrete, holistic concept. The proposed conceptual model which then emerged provides a concrete, testable framework for caring in nursing.

The model has been supported through student analyses at both the doctoral and master's levels in nursing using Fawcett's (1984) criteria for conceptual model evaluation (Ingle, 1987a; Burns, 1989; Jordan, 1989). Finally, the model was adopted as the Conceptual Framework for a National League for Nursing-accredited Upper Division Baccalaureate Nursing Program (BSN Program Self-Study, Vermont College of Norwich University, 1990).

This proposed model both draws from and extends Mayeroff's (1971) philosophical notion of human caring, Gaut's (1979, 1981, 1983, 1984a, 1984b) philosophical analysis of intentional caring in nursing, and Watson's (1979, 1985) model of caring as therapeutic interpersonal process in nursing. The following discussion will present the proposed model within the context of points of agreement and contrast with its philosophic antecedents. Expansion beyond these antecedents will be discussed in the presentation of the conceptual model.

CARING'S ANTECEDENT CONCEPTUALIZATION:
A REVIEW OF SELECTED RELATED LITERATURE

Mayeroff's (1971) eight ingredients of human caring include: knowing, alternating rhythms, patience, honesty, trust, courage, humility, and hope. These ingredients comprise the caring process which inevitably helps the carer to grow toward self-actualization. According to Mayeroff, the caring process rather than its action bestows self-meaning, thereby giving meaning to one's life. This model supports Mayeroff's work insofar as caring is conceptualized as a process central to nursing practice.

Gaut's (1979, 1981, 1983, 1984a, 1984b) model of caring in nursing was seminal to the development of the following conceptual model, which expands on her philosophic analysis of caring as intentional action. Gaut's work builds on that of Kerr and Soltis (1974), who described a model of intentional action in education. Gaut's (1981) model also evolved in large part from the work of earlier nurse scholars. These included Nightingale (1969), Paterson and Zderad (1976), Leininger (1977), Bevis (1978), and Watson (1979). Nonnurse scholars whose ideas influenced Gaut's work included Marcel (1964, 1967), Teilhard de Chardin (1967), Rollo May (1969), Buber (1970), Mayeroff (1971), and Maslow (1975).

Gaut asserts that professional caring in nursing is operationally different from natural caring. Her central thesis of caring as a concept in nursing recognizes caring's biological, psychological, and emotional components. Caring occurs indirectly through other activities. As such, caring is "mediated action" (Gaut, 1979, p. 120). An action is caring if the carer's intention, action, and situation context are purposefully organized around the concept of caring. Gaut (1979, 1981, 1983, 1984a) asserts that her's is a purely action model.

Watson (1979, 1985) views caring in nursing as both humanistic and scientific. Caring is a process which uses caring methods to bring about health which is positive. This process includes the use of therapeutic interpersonal interchange between nurse and patient. Extending Nodding's (1984) view of caring as feminine, Watson (1989) asserts that the female-dominated nursing profession "can more clearly . . . call forth a model of human centeredness and subjectivity" than is feasible from the male-dominated medical profession (p. 127). Watson's vision of nurse caring as therapeutic interpersonal process supported the development of the following proposed conceptual model.

THE CONCEPTUAL MODEL

This proposed conceptual model connects direct caring action(s) in nursing to an intentionally caring process. The model thus extends Gaut's conceptualization of caring as indirect action only (Gaut, 1979, 1981, 1983, 1984a). Building on the idea of an enfolding universe (Bohm, 1957, 1978, 1980), professional nurse caring conceptually enfolds rather than differs from natural caring.

This conceptual model uses Bohm's (1957) second model of undivided wholeness in an attempt to overcome language constraints inherent in discussing a holistic worldview. Bohm states that his model demonstrates wholeness as flowing movement. He exemplifies wholeness as a drop of dye added to a viscous liquid like glycerine, contained between two glass cylinders. The outer glass cylinder is slowly rotated, during which the drop of dye flows out into the glycerine. Following several cylinder rotations, the dye is no longer discretely apparent. Its essence is no longer explicit within the glycerine. Were the cylinder to be slowly rotated in the opposite direction the same number of rotations, however, the dye's hidden essence would again become implicit. In this way, Bohm (1978) asserts that hidden essence, or order, flows throughout the whole. As such, this wholeness constitutes an implicate ordering of the universe.

The idea that professional nurse caring is holistic cannot be conveyed as a whole through the single mode of language. The hologram, therefore, can serve as a visual metaphor for the conceptual model of professional nurse caring. Watson (1986) was the first to use the hologram in order to visually describe caring's holism. A hologram can reproduce the whole within any one part, however small. As a hologram, then, professional nurse caring is what it is, whole and entire. Its practice requires that the nurse address the *whole* client.

The concept of professional caring provides a vision for nursing around which practice, education, administration, and research can be organized, and a conceptual model for nursing can be developed. The following model as tested suggests that professional nurse caring may delineate a practice area for nursing, at least in the United States (Hernandez, 1985, 1987, 1988, 1989, in press; Ingle, 1987b; Burns, under investigation).

Definitions

In discussing the practice of nursing based on the concept of professional caring, the following definitions are fundamental to this conceptual model:

> *Professional caring as intentional action:* within the scope of this proposed conceptual model, all nursing therapeutics encompass intentional caring action. Nursing's professional intentional actions are professionally learned through formal education in nursing as well as through professional role-modeling and experience. Intentional caring action in nursing differs from that of other professions as well as from natural human caring because of this learning. The "development of natural capacities [for caring] . . . and acquired modifications of such natural capacities" nevertheless must underpin the nurse's intentional practice of professional nurse caring (Gustafson, 1981, p. 43).

> *Natural caring:* a human process and activity wherein one assists another in growth and actualization. Giving caring to another in turn can potentiate one's self-actualization (Mayeroff, 1971).

> *Professional nurse caring:* operationally enfolds natural caring, and can only be taught to nurses following or concurrent with their

living the experience of natural caring. Professional nurse caring is learned and transmitted with therapeutic intent as a direct nursing intervention. The nurse intentionally uses professional caring as the *modus* or therapeutic means for meeting a client's assessed needs, in order to attain nursing and client health care goals (Hernandez, 1989, in press). The sustenance for such caring arises from *client* practice, but must also derive from its *collegial* practice (Hernandez, 1989). Within the context of this model, the client can be an individual, group (either related or not), or a population. The client is the coparticipant in nursing care.

Collegial caring: coexistent with the nurse's practice of client-centered professional caring, collegial caring can provide actualization to the nurse who otherwise may perceive either diminished or absent actualization in giving professional caring to clients. Such actualization can be fostered because the process of collegial caring includes the implication that the nurse will experience reciprocation of that caring. That is, a professional environment organized around this conceptual model is one in which caring given is also caring received.

Agency, Patiency, and Goals

Nursing is both the process and the action of professional nurse caring, wherein the nurse coparticipates with the client as a whole in implementing the nursing process. The primary focus of professional nurse caring is direct, intentional, and therapeutic involvement with the client. In addition, each individual is a unique being who interacts–interfaces as one with the environment communicating with, responding to, and impacting both self and others. Human beings are but one explication of the environment, however. Cognizant of this environmental inclusivity and of each human's individuality, the nurse involves the client (an individual or group, either related or not; or a population) in using the nursing process to assess, plan, implement, and evaluate care directed toward meeting identified needs.

Health is an ongoing process. Health's focus is positive. Nursing's health goal is one of helping the client to achieve optimum wellness or death with dignity.

Assumptions

Although a collegial caring environment is fundamental to the practice of professional nurse caring, a pre-nursing natural caring experiential grounding must underpin the nurse's practice of professional caring. This lived experience can also be provided or supplemented during the education process in nursing. Three basic assumptions thus frame this conceptual model:

1. The capacity to give and receive caring is a natural ability.

2. The nurse's ability to practice professional caring is predicated on the nurse achieving the lived experience of self-actualizing natural caring.

3. The nurse cares for and respects his or her own self.

Propositions

Five propositions organize this conceptual model. They reflect the philosophic as well as research perspectives which contributed to the model's development and refinement (Gustafson, 1981; Rosenthal & Bourgeois, 1983; Hernandez, 1987, 1988a, 1989; Ingle, 1987b). These propositions stipulate that the practice of professional caring requires the nurse to:

1. Participate in collegial caring activities (e.g., staff meetings and formal/informal support groups) in order to facilitate self-actualization.

2. Believe in the value of professional nurse caring.

3. Have the desire to act.

4. Know that one will intentionally act.

5. Recognize that professional nurse caring is a process that can be directly and intentionally communicated.

Requirements for the Practice of
Professional Nurse Caring

As stated earlier, the natural caring experience is foundational to the nurse's ability to practice professional caring. The lived experience of natural caring provides the nurse with the readiness to practice professional nurse caring, predicated upon meeting three conditions:

1. The nurse must learn both *how* and *how best* to transmit professional caring. This learning can occur through a variety of ways, including both formal and informal education as well as exposure to and practice of caring.

2. The nurse must be technically competent. Achieving psychomotor technical competence leads to *feeling* competent. With

the eventual added dimension of collegial validation of this competence, the nurse will experience the empowerment and self-actualization derived from giving professional caring.

3. The nurse must achieve professional confidence. Professional confidence is closely allied both to *learning* as well as to *technical competence*. The give and take of professional experience as well as collegial and client validation of nursing skills enable the nurse to work with clients in a professional caring and therapeutic manner.

These conditions need not be met simultaneously or in any particular order of cognitive/psychomotor/affective attainment. They are not hierarchical in terms of achieving expertise in professional caring. These three conditions can be summarized heuristically as:

LEARNING + COMPETENCE + CONFIDENCE = CARING CAPABILITY

Learning how to practice professional nurse caring as well as gaining technical competence and professional confidence facilitate the development of a caring behavioral repertoire. The three interpersonal communicators of touching, listening, and verbal–nonverbal communication can directly and intentionally transmit professional nurse caring. Such caring supports client self-actualization. As Larsen (1981) asserts, the nurse–client relationship is generally secondary to the primary relationship the client experiences with significant others. Nurse self-actualization experienced as a result of caring for the client thus may not always occur. Benner (1984, 1988) states that one cannot command caring—one can only strive to understand and so enable caring's occurrence. Within the context of this conceptual model, then, nurse self-actualization may not derive from every client caring encounter. (Nevertheless, the nurse should strive to facilitate such self-actualization through its engenderment with the client.) When caring is perceived as coming back to the nurse in the course of giving caring to a client, the nurse is coactualized. As a necessary adjunct to such coactualizing experiences, collegial relationships provide a rich source for the reciprocation of caring which is integral to nurse self-actualization.

THE CONCEPTUAL MODEL'S VISION
OF THE CARING PROCESS

Seven subconcepts guide the textual explication of professional nurse caring. Figure 1 presents a schematic model of these concepts.

Figure 1
The Seven Sub-Concepts of
Professional Nurse Caring

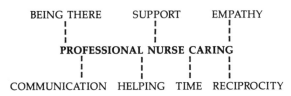

Being there for the client provides comfort and security. It can be both verbally and nonverbally expressed, but is dependent upon the nurse's *demonstrated, predictable,* and *nonjudgmental* presence for the client. In this way the nurse transmits *support* through providing nurturance, advocacy via reliable alliance, and health information access. Such involvement requires that the nurse have empathy for the client. *Empathy* derives from life experience and as such enables the nurse to understand and accept the client—in other words, to enter into the client's reality—without attempting to influence or change the client.

Professional nurse caring is transmitted to others through interpersonal *communication.* This communication can be verbal or nonverbal. Touching can be a powerful mode for communicating professional nurse caring. Through being there for the client, while using the empathic self to communicate support, the nurse can effectively help the client to attain health or care delivery goals. *Helping* others requires that the nurse perceive that *time* is available to practice caring. Within this model, the practice of professional nursing is holistic. Lack of time can reduce nursing's practice to delivery of technical tasks, thus negating nursing's holistic practice.

In order to maintain or recharge one's caring capacity, the nurse must feel that his or her practice of professional caring with clients as well as colleagues is reciprocated. *Reciprocity* of caring is thus fundamental to the nurse's practice of professional caring, because it is through caring's reciprocation that the nurse can achieve self-actualization. Client reciprocation of caring may not always occur. In addition, client caring may not always lead the nurse to experience the self-actualization needed to gain or maintain the psychic energy required to continue to give professional caring. Therefore, the nurse can also achieve actualization through giving and receiving professional caring from colleagues. If a nurse is not perceived by colleagues as both technically competent and professionally confident, however, professional

Figure 2
Schema of the Proposed Conceptual Model of Professional Nurse Caring

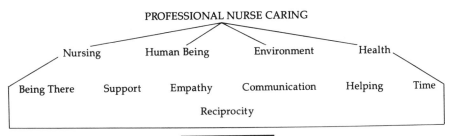

PROFESSIONAL NURSE CARING

Nursing   Human Being   Environment   Health

Being There   Support   Empathy   Communication   Helping   Time

Reciprocity

caring's reciprocation may be compromised. In other words, through providing for professional self-actualization, collegially-experienced professional nurse caring can both validate nursing practice as well as provide the psychic energy necessary to the nurse's continued ability to transmit professional caring to clients. This is especially true in those scenarios where the nurse is unable to engender client acknowledgment that caring was either received or valued.

Collegial participation in professional nurse caring is more than a benefit of practicing nursing using this model. That is, the nurse's fundamental ability to practice professional caring with the client depends on the experience of professional caring with colleagues. (Such caring can be expressed, for example, in the respect of one colleague for another.) As an adjunct to natural caring the nurse might experience in personal life, professional caring practiced with colleagues can facilitate that self-actualization which is a necessary concomitant to the caring process.

Figure 2 illustrates the foregoing conceptual model in only one dimension. It is not technically feasible to present a metaphor for the model as a hologram. The reader is, therefore, asked to creatively visualize this schema as a holistic, multidimensional reality.

CONCLUSION

This conceptual model can expand some of the existing thought on caring. It offers rich possibilities for testing the full range of nursing's uniqueness and its practice. In the final analysis, research is beginning to support the idea that caring formulates more than nursing's essence. That is, nursing (may) = professional nurse caring.

REFERENCES

Benner, P. (1984). *From novice to expert.* Menlo Park, CA: Addison-Wesley.

Benner, P. (1988). *The primacy of caring: Stress and coping in health and illness.* Menlo Park, CA: Addison-Wesley.

Bevis, E. O. (1978). *Curriculum building in nursing: A process.* (2nd ed.). St. Louis: C.V. Mosby.

Bohm, D. (1957). *Causality and chance in modern physics.* London: Routledge & Kegan Paul.

Bohm, D. (1978). The enfolding-unfolding universe: An interview with R. Weber. *Revision, 1*(3-4), 24-51.

Bohm, D. (1980). *Wholeness and the implicate order.* London: Routledge & Kegan Paul.

Buber, M. (1970). *I and thou* (W. Kaufman, trans.). New York: Charles Scribner's Sons.

de Chardin, T. (1967). *On love.* Pittsburgh: Duquesne University Press.

Burns, E. (1989). *Watson's and Hernandez' theories of nurse caring: A comparative analysis.* Unpublished master's paper. The Graduate Program in the School of Professional Nursing, The University of Vermont.

Burns, E. (under investigation). *A qualitative investigation of nurses' perceptions of their practice professional nurse caring in a critical care unit.* Unpublished master's thesis proposal. The Graduate Program in Nursing, The University of Vermont.

Fawcett, J. (1984). *Analysis and evaluation of conceptual models of nursing.* Philadelphia: F.A. Davis.

Gaut, D. A. (1979). *An application of the Kerr-Soltis model to the concept of caring in nursing education.* Unpublished doctoral dissertation. University of Washington.

Gaut, D. A. (1981). Conceptual analysis of caring: Research method. In M. M. Leininger (Ed.), *Caring: An essential human need.* Thorofare, NJ: Slack.

Gaut, D. A. (1983). Development of a theoretically adequate description of caring. *Western Journal of Nursing Research, 5*(4), 313-324.

Gaut, D. A. (1984a). A philosophic orientation to caring research. In M. M. Leininger (Ed.), *Care: The essence of nursing and health.* Thorofare, NJ: Slack.

Gaut, D. A. (1984b). A theoretic description of caring as action. In M. M. Leininger (Ed.), *Care: The essence of nursing and health*. Thorofare, NJ: Slack.

Gilligan, C. (1982). *In a different voice: Psychological theory and women's development*. Cambridge: Harvard University Press.

Gustafson, D. (1981). Passivity and activity in intentional actions. *Mind, 90*, 41–60.

Hernandez, C. M. (1985). *A conceptualization of professional nurse caring in community health nurses: A qualitative investigation*. Unpublished doctoral research. Adelphi University.

Hernandez, C. M. G. (1987). *A phenomenologic investigation of the concept of the lived experience of caring in professional nurses*. Unpublished doctoral dissertation. Adelphi University.

Hernandez, C. M. G. (1988a). *A phenomenologic investigation of the lived experience of caring in technical nurses*. Unpublished research.

Hernandez, C. G. (1988b). Professional nurse caring: A proposed model for nursing. In Igoe, J., Reeder, F., Sakalys, J., Webster, D., et al (Eds.), *Conference Proceedings: Caring and Nursing in the Feminist Perspectives*. Denver: School of Nursing, University of Colorado.

Hernandez, C. G. (1989). Caring as a paradigm for nursing. *Conference Proceedings: International Council of Nurses, 19th Quadrennial Seoul Congress*. Seoul, Korea; and *Conference Proceedings: Advances in International Nursing Scholarship, Sigma Theta Tau International Research Congress*, Taipei, Taiwan.

Hernandez, C. G. (in press). Caring as a lived experience in professional nurses: A phenomenologic investigation. In P. Chinn (Ed.), *An anthology of caring*. New York: National League for Nursing.

Ingle, J. (1987a). *Evaluation of a theoretical model for nursing science: Hernandez's conceptual model of caring*. Unpublished doctoral paper. The School of Nursing in the Graduate School, The University of Alabama at Birmingham.

Ingle, J. (1987b). *Utilization in nursing practice of Hernandez's conceptual model of caring*. Unpublished doctoral research. The School of Nursing in the Graduate School, The University of Alabama at Birmingham.

Ingle, J. (1988). *The business of caring: The perspective of men in nursing*. Unpublished doctoral dissertation. The School of Nursing in the Graduate School, the University of Alabama at Birmingham.

Jordan, S. (1989). *An analysis of Hernandez's theoretical framework of professional nurse caring.* Unpublished master's paper. The Graduate Program in the School of Professional Nursing, The University of Vermont.

Kerr, D. H., & Soltis, J. F. (1974). Locating teacher competency: An action description of teaching. *Educational Therapy, 24*(1), 3–16.

Larsen, P. J. (1981). *Oncology patients' and professional nurses' perceptions of important nurse caring behaviors.* Unpublished doctoral dissertation. University of California at San Francisco.

Leininger, M. M. (1977). The phenomenon of caring: The essence and central focus of nursing. *American Nurses Foundation* (Nursing Research Report), *12*(1), 2, 14.

Marcel, G. (1964). *Creative fidelity* (R. Rosthal, trans.). New York: The Monday Press.

Marcel, G. (1967). *Presence and immortality.* Pittsburgh: Duquesne University Press.

Maslow, A. (1975). Love in healthy people. In A. Montague (Ed.), *The Practice of Love.* Englewood Cliffs, NJ: Prentice-Hall.

May, R. (1969). *Love and will.* New York: W.W. Norton.

Mayeroff, M. (1971). *On caring.* New York: Harper and Row.

Nightingale, F. (1969). Notes on nursing. New York: Dover Publications.

Noddings, N. (1984). *Caring: A feminine approach to ethics and moral education.* Berkeley: University of California Press.

Paterson, J., & Zderad, L. (1976). *Humanistic nursing.* New York: John Wiley, and Sons.

Rosenthal, S. B., & Bourgeois, P. I. (1983). Lewis, Heidegger and ontological presence. *Philosophy Today, 27*(4), 290–296.

Watson, J. (1979). *Nursing: The philosophy and science of caring.* Boston: Little, Brown.

Watson, J. (1985). *Nursing: Human science and human care. A theory of nursing.* Norwalk, CT: Appleton-Century-Crofts.

Watson, J. (1986). Formal presentation, first annual nurse scholar lecture. New York: Columbia University.

Watson, J. (1989). Human caring and suffering: A subjective model for health sciences. In R. L. Taylor & J. Watson (Eds.), *They shall not hurt.* Boulder: Colorado University Press.

9

Gender and Cost in Caring

Debbie Ward

Caring *is* work. Yet the two concepts lie an uneasy distance from one another. Caring is widely seen as private and sacrificial nurturing, but not demanding labor. Work is public and paid exertion, and not the stuff of an expressive relationship between caregiver and care recipient. The distance between the two concepts of caring and work is a gap straddled daily by nurses. This paper presents some initial considerations on the nature of the gap and reflects my interest in the labor of nursing.

One way to think about caring as work is to look at its value. What is caregiving worth? And how should we determine its value? Nursing is at work on detailing the stuff of caring. Scholars and researchers are looking at the attitudes of the cared-for and the caregivers. They are looking at the psychological burdens and benefits of caring. But the language of psychological attitudes and individual behavior does not tell all nor does it speak to everybody about caring. I am interested in using language to describe the work of caring that most people understand: time and money.

My doctoral work was in health policy, and my dissertation was on caring for the frail elderly at home by family members and friends. At the outset, I rejected the commonly used term "family care." The work of caregiving is not done by all family members; most of it is done by women. I used the term "kin care," adapting the term from the work of the anthropologist Michaela di Leonardo (1984). In *Varieties of Ethnic Experience*, di Leonardo wrote about *kin work*—the work done almost exclusively by women maintaining the

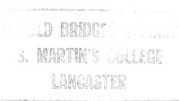

family network. I know each of you has done some of this work—
transmitting news or carrying out a family ritual from an elaborate Thanksgiv-
ing meal to buying the right kind of pajamas.

Di Leonardo's term struck me. These family-maintaining activities are *work*:
"bodily or mental effort exerted to do or make something; purposeful activity."
(Webster's New Universal Unabridged Dictionary, Second edition, 1983). But
we don't think of kin work in this way. Di Leonardo recently wrote a piece
on the female work of card-giving and organizing remembrances. I would guess
that most of us, in thinking about a trip to buy a card to give to someone, would
not classify this activity as work.

But why not?

There are several reasons. But among them are two important and related
reasons:

1. The activity is unpaid.
2. The activity is done by women.

The paradigmatic case of unpaid activity by women is housework. My
interest in care of the frail elderly as a piece of homework in particular was
long preceded by my interest in housework as a category in general. The
classic piece of feminist work, *The Politics of Housework*, by Pam Mainairdi in
the late 1960s, is a call to revolution, forcing the entry of men into the realm of
housework. Dating from the "Aha" experience of reading Mainairdi (and
probably actually much earlier from my hatred of repetitive household labor
such as setting the table only to clear it again reinforced with the guilt of
seeing everyone's mother including my own labor endlessly in the Sisyphean
household for the benefit of spouse and offspring), I have always wondered
why the work surrounding families and home falls to women. I understand
that only women birth babies. I continue to wonder why only women do
housework. So when my dissertation topic moved toward care of the elderly,
it quickly became clear that I would look at caregiver work.

But it was luck, not forethought, that brought me an article by the British
scholar, Janet Finch, on the extent of caregiving work done by women in
Great Britain. (The bibliographic kindness of friends in leading me to Finch's
work points up what is wrongly seen as a curse for nursing: the interdisciplinary nature of our scholarship. Without the broadening influence of fields
such as sociology, economics, and particularly women's studies, nursing would
suffer.) Friends led me first to Janet Finch's work and then to a particular
article in the British journal, *Radical Community Medicine*, in which Finch
did an enlightening thing. She determined how many hours British women
spent caring for disabled and ill family members and multiplied those hours by

the median wage at the time. She came up with a figure that surpassed the entire National Health Service budget.

I used Finch's example to analyze care of the frail elderly in the United States. I took the essential form of unpaid caring—family maintenance or housework—as a model. I looked at gender and cost in kin care, using historical, political, sociological, and economic work done on housework as a guide.

Like other forms of household work, kin care is overwhelmingly the work of women. And like other forms of household work, it is popularly regarded as a free good. In the same way that calculating the value of housework into the Gross National Product points out a hole in the standard method of valuing national goods and services, assigning dollar value to unpaid caring forces a new look at the undervalued labor of kin care. When caring is removed from the realm of "sacrifice" and "duty" and examined with dollar signs, its gender asymmetry takes on new meaning.

I computed the value of the hours spent in caregiving, based on a 1982 national survey of caregivers to the frail elderly (Stone et al, 1986). Seventy-two percent of the respondent caregivers were women. They provided elder care on average four hours a day. Over three-quarters (78.9%) of the sample provided care seven days a week. Extrapolating from the sample to a population estimated at 2.2 million caregivers, it could be estimated that 2,712,160,000 hours of caregiving work were contributed without pay in 1982. If you apply some simple and straightforward multipliers to calculate the value of those hours, you come up with some very big numbers.

For example, if you use the minimum wage—$3.35 an hour in 1982 until it was raised to $3.80 in April 1990—the value of that year's worth of care was $9,860,736,000.00.

If you use the hourly wage of a home health aide—estimated at $4—the value of that year's worth of care was $10,848,640,000.00.

If you use home health aid *charges*—that is, what someone would have had to pay to buy those hours of care at a very conservative price of $6.50 an hour—the value of that care comes to $17,629,040,000.00.

This 17.6 billion dollar figure—the replacement cost for a year of unpaid caregiving—is greater than the 1982 federal budget for Medicare payments for medical (not hospital) services. In 1982, 15.5 billion dollars were paid for care to over 25 million enrollees over age 65. Seventeen billion dollars in unpaid home caregiving is almost half the budget-breaking federal Medicare payment in 1982 to hospitals, some 35 billion dollars ($35,631,000,000). Even the lowest value calculated for unpaid kin care far exceeded the 1982 federal reimbursement to home health vendors, a paltry 496 million dollars.

The staggering amounts I calculated certainly do *not* approximate the total value of the labor contributed by caregivers. For each caregiver's total contribution we would have to compute many additional costs: her costs if she bought replacement services, her loss in wages if she had to cut back on work, her pension loss, her losses from foregone promotions and advancement, retraining costs if she re-entered work at a later time, loss in benefits, the value of her lost leisure time, and the value of items she may have purchased in order to do the caregiving work or of the income support she provided to the cared-for persons.

So the amounts calculated for the group are clearly underestimates. Nonetheless, they represent a range of what I characterize as a *subsidy to the social welfare*, paid by caregivers, primarily women, who give their time and labor.

Caregivers contribute a service that has value—yet one that is still labeled "free." Caregivers of both genders will pay these socially invisible costs. But clearly women are the group most affected. They experience disproportionate costs having to do with caregiving.

Evidence supports the disproportionate economic burden born by women in a wide variety of caregiving situations, not just those having to do with elder care. Economist Heidi Hartmann, testifying before a Senate subcommittee considering parental leave legislation, reported a study using data from the Panel Study of Income Dynamics. Nearly 7,000 families in this long-running study are interviewed yearly on multiple issues having to do with work and family. Hartmann and her colleagues compared women under 41 years of age with a serious attachment to the workforce who had a baby with those women who did not have a child. They compared women with and without some form of employment leave, and they compared women with new babies with men with new babies.

It is this last comparison on which I will dwell. Using two indicators, hourly wages and hours of housework (not including hours spent on child-care), women are shown to bear a disproportionate share of the costs of having children.

> While the differences between women and men are substantial in the year before the birth, they are greatly magnified subsequent to a birth (or adoption). By two years after the birth, women's wages relative to men's have declined by 60 percent (in constant dollars) and their housework hours have increased 22 percent. Thus, as a result of having a baby, economic equity between the sexes declines, and women become increasingly burdened with unpaid work. Other researchers have shown that this uneven exchange will go on to have negative consequences for women's lifetime earnings and even for their retirement income and economic status in old age. (Hartmann, 1978, pp. 7–8)

The Family Survival Project in San Francisco works with families providing long-term care for their chronically impaired, often traumatically brain-injured, members. The Project found that employed caregivers (N = 143, 70 + % were female) worked as many hours caregiving as they did at paid work—roughly 35 hours per week (Petty & Friss, 1987).

What do such studies tell us about caregiving? We already knew that most caregiving, both paid and unpaid, falls to women. We learned that the extent of unpaid caregiving work is enormous, and when assigned value in the form of dollars is a massive contribution. Hartmann's work tells us that taking on the most routine caregiving responsibilities—for example, child care—causes a significant decline in lifetime earnings. The family survival study as well as the numbers I've reviewed show that caregiving is another full-time job. These data are essential to understanding women's baseline economic disadvantage and the cycle of poverty in which many women, especially single mothers, are trapped.

Now that we've looked at the economics of caregiving, the question about housework that plagued me is restated: Why does this costly labor fall to women?

The answers to this question range across women's history, from the cult of domesticity which idealized women's role at home to the remarkable lack of development of appropriate household technology. In this forum I can only point to some of the effects of allocating work by gender. Caregiving roles are both idealized by society as, at the same time, they serve to isolate women from "real life." "Women are socialized to a value system of responsiveness and care that is antithetical to marketplace norms of competition and financial gain. They are expected to perform unpaid work that underpins the economy yet is peripheral to the economy as defined by men." (Hooyman & Ryan, 1987, p. 170.)

Where do nurses stand in an environment so constrained that women are obligated to do work that is not valued? As is true for women's work in general, overall wages for nurses have been low. And like all women, nurses do double duty—full-time work at the work site and at home. Double duty is becoming the norm for white women of all classes, as it has always been for women of color and poor women. More than half of new mothers of all races are remaining in the work force.

But nurses are in a peculiar situation in which the work they do at home and the work they do on the job have great similarities. They do caregiving work for which they are both paid and unpaid. Recent developments in health care in the United States point up some of the special tensions of nurses' work. One such development is the shortened length of hospital stays.

Sociologist Nona Glazer, writing on women health workers, asks—when home care is extolled as a virtue and backed up by early discharge from hospital, who does the recuperative, supervisory work at home? Women. So nurses who run day surgeries and release children home after two hours are in effect turning over their once paid-for labor to their unpaid sisters. A nurse herself might forego a day's salary to stay home to nurse a recuperating child. "Health care has always been done in the home by wives and mothers, and daughters and daughters-in-law. Women's work in the home expands, however, with shortened hospital stays, increased outpatient clinic treatment, less paid professional and technical nursing, and more home care" (Glazer, 1988, p. 130). Most health workers and insurers once opposed home care but increasingly home care is being supported by professional groups as long as those groups have authority to supervise that care. Nurses may not see that increased calls for care at home also mean increased work shifted to "the private family and the isolated woman within it. . . . New health policies . . . rest on women picking up the newly unpaid work, accepting the increased domestic work that results from the decommodification (transfer of work from paid to unpaid workers) of hospital labor, for discharge planners, home care supervisors, and insurers expect these women to do the work of caring for those with acute and chronic medical problems" (Glazer, p. 131).

Glazer (1984) draws an interesting parallel with what happened to retail work—shoppers became their own clerks, thereby increasing profits for owners and managers. "The retail trade analogue of early patient discharge, outpatient treatment, and self-care by family members is self-service by shoppers" (Glazer, 1988, p. 134). This shift of caring labor from workplace to home has affected members of different economic classes differently. Those who are able to, pay for substitute labor. Those who cannot, fit in the additional work as they are able. Few nurses could afford to purchase home nursing, especially if they are sole providers for a household.

I think it's useful for all of us as women—and particularly as nurses—to think about our paid and unpaid caregiving and recognize the *fact* of double duty. Lawyer Mary Frances Berry, speaking at the 1987 National Women's Studies Association meeting at Spelman College in Atlanta, Georgia, said that economic and policy reforms won't mean much for women's status as long as they remain the primary caretakers. "Until roles change, women are fools to want to be treated equally without help." Our unpaid work, alone and in combination with unequally compensated paid labor, is a subsidy women provide to the general social welfare.

I'm advocating an expanded view of caring in which it is honored, not cheapened, by assigning monetary value. In my view, caregivers would demand valuation of their time, rather than demur with protestations that their time is worthless. From this point of view, one might speculate that hurried hospital discharges and reduced nursing home beds have among their many effects an increase in the unpaid labor of wives, daughters, grandmothers, and other women who find they are obligated to do caregiving work for free. Where might this broadened view of women's work lead nurses?

In the short term, until publicly supported caregiving is adequately funded, we can insist that caregiving not be entirely women's work. Both men and women must be convinced of this.

And we have to help women assess whether they are able to take on caregiving work in addition to normal family work. Rather than assuming that women will automatically absorb any additional caregiving work, we might start by exploring options with caregivers. The introduction of the topic may be difficult, as an article in the social work literature suggests.

> *Unhappily, many caregivers may neither gratefully nor eagerly accept such interventions [assessing caregiver ability and desire]. Many do not perceive their circumstances as extraordinary; a sense of selflessness and duty often overrides their sense of personal hazard. Some caregivers do not attribute their distress to the untenable situations they face, but rather to their inability to cope. Thus, in addition to locating resources and making referrals, the social worker may need to provide reassurance and support to caregivers who feel that using outside resources is an admission of failure.* (p. 28)

It is an accepted standard of excellent nursing care that nurses promote realistic assessments. They do not falsely reassure—"Everything's going to be fine." Instead they promote optimum coping—"Soon you will be taking excellent care of your colostomy on your own." Applying the same standard, nurses evaluating home care situations need to discuss the economic consequences of choosing to provide kin care.

In the long term, many important efforts come to mind which may shape caregiving. The improvement of institutions and agency care, of course, marks an important beginning. A caregiver says "I can't put him in an institution." What if institutions were excellent places in which to live? ". . . [T]he failures of institutions, which have resulted in accelerated community and home-based care, place additional burden on women caregivers." (Briar & Ryan, 1986, p. 31.) What if women—nurses and caregivers—designed, ran, and set policy for institutions?

Another important effort is to ensure adequate reimbursement for long-term care. Nurses and caregivers, understanding the value of their work, may yet successfully lobby for a shift in the national accounting such that services to the growing population of elderly are valued at least as highly as acute inpatient care.

In looking ahead to the future of women's work, I'll add one last caveat. Expanded services and adequate financial support will help resolve the long-term care crisis, but I believe we need to step back far enough to worry about the push to "help women balance work and family" and ask why women should do all the balancing. I have a particular worry about the long-term effects of flex-time and other benefits for women. I think we may thereby create what I call the "organizational menstrual hut," a confine for women wherein they can work hard and enjoy each other's company but from which they do not get the major promotions nor the benefits from full equality in the work place.

And while we're stepping back for the long view, let's remember that the lessons on the precarious economic straits of women are not only for patients—they are for us, nurses working and growing old. As caregivers and as workers, we need to agitate for economic security through a variety of mechanisms: the institution of career ladders in nursing, adequate retirement income, and funded day care for children and adults, including sick child care. We have a lot of work to do; let's be sure it all gets counted.

REFERENCES

Berry, M. F. (1987, August). *off our backs, 17*(8), 21.

Briar, K. H., & R. Ryan. (1986, spring). The anti-institution movement and women caregivers. *Affilia, 5*(2), 20–31.

di Leonardo, M. (1984). *Varieties of ethnic experience.* Ithaca, NY: Cornell University Press.

di Leonardo, M. (1987). The female world of cards and holidays. *Signs 12*(3), 440–453.

Finch, J. (1976, summer). Community care and the invisible welfare state. *Radical Community Medicine,* 15–21.

Glazer, N. (1984). Servants to capital: Unpaid domestic labor and paid work. *Revue of Radical Political Economics, 16*(1), 61–87.

Glazer, N. (1988). Overlooked, overworked: Women's unpaid and paid work in the health services "cost crisis." *International Journal of Health Services, 18*(1), 119–137.

Hartmann, H. (1987). Testimony to the Senate Subcommittee on Children, Families, Drugs and Alcoholism. October 29, 1987.

Hooyman, N. R., & R. Ryan. (1987) Women as caregivers of the elderly: Catch-22 dilemmas. In J. Figueira-McDonough & R. Sarri (Eds.). *The* trapped woman. Human Services Series Sourcebook Volume IV. Beverly Hills, CA: Sage, pp. 143–171.

Mainairdi, P. undated pamphlet. *The Politics of Housework.*

Petty, D., & L. Friss. (1987, October) A balancing act of working and caregiving. *Business and Health* 4(12), 22–26.

Stone, R. et al. (1986). *Caregivers of the frail elderly: A national profile.* Rockville, Maryland: Division of Intramural Research, National Center for Health Services Research and Health Care Technology Assessment.

Ward, D. (1987). *The new old burden: Gender and cost in kin care of disabled elderly.* Doctoral Dissertation. Boston University, Boston, Massachusetts.

10

Intersubjective Copresence in a Caring Model

Sharon Horner

This model focuses on the caring that occurs between nurses and clients. Pellegrino (1985) identified the traditional forms of caring in the health professions as follows: (1) compassion, or feeling the client's pain; (2) performing activities of daily living when the client is unable to do so; (3) taking over problem solving for the client; and (4) carrying out technical procedures. In the face of increasing complaints from consumers about the lack of caring they receive, one must question which form of caring is missing?

THEORETICAL OVERVIEW

Since early in this century, nurses have increased their proficiency in technical skills (Reverby, 1987) in congruence with Pellegrino's model of caring. However, with higher technical skills comes the dehumanization of the client: treating the respirator and Swan-Ganz catheter rather than the human being in the bed (Carper, 1986).

Caring is that relationship in which feelings of concern, regard, or respect of one human being for another are expressed (Boyle, 1981). It occurs in interactions when each person is perceived to be a unique, genuinely feeling and reacting being (Gadow, 1985; Paulen & Rapp, 1981). In professional caring, it is desirable for the nurse to interact with the client as an individual while at the same time delivering knowledgeable, skilled care (Boyle, 1981). In Pellegrino's (1985) classification, however, only compassion reflects this concern for the client's subjective experiences.

Gadow (1985) states that caring is purposeful: It is directed toward the achievement of goals identified by the client with assistance from the nurse. Mayeroff (1971) states that in caring there is mutual self-actualization, toward which both parties are striving through their interactions.

It has been proposed that nursing should provide caring to all clients. Yet caring involves more than caretaking, or technical skills. Interpersonal interactions that reflect an understanding of the client's subjective experiences are paramount. Unfortunately, it is not possible to share the subjective experiences of all clients one comes in contact with. As a result, universality of caring becomes extremely difficult, if possible at all (Noddings, 1984).

In order to care, one must perceive the other as a unique being and be open to the other's subjective interpretations and experiences of events while supporting the other's attainment of certain agreed on goals. Key concepts in this model include caring, perception, humanistic goals, and intersubjective copresence.

DEFINITIONS OF CONCEPTS

Caring

According to Webster's Unabridged Dictionary, *caring* is defined as mental pain, anxiety, solicitude, watchfulness, or inclination for something or someone (McKechnie, 1983). This definition indicates the feeling state associated with caring; however, the professional person who demonstrates caring is involved in more than a feeling response to another's situation, the professional must *act* on the other's behalf. Leininger (1981) defines caring as those assistive, supportive, or facilitative acts directed toward another, in order to improve or to maintain a favorably healthy condition for life.

Noddings (1984) writes that the action component of caring may be an overt behavioral response, but there are times when the act is one of commitment to another. For example, there are many situations when a person does not need to have something done for him or her, but requires the assurance that there is someone who supports his or her decisions, or his or her view of self. In this model, caring becomes a complex interpersonal interaction between a nurse and client, in which each perceives the other as a unique responsive individual, and which incorporates both feeling and behavioral, or commitment, responses which are directed toward humanistic goals.

Intersubjective Copresence

Caring interactions are enhanced when one perceives the reality of the other or views the world through the other's eyes, and then acts accordingly, from a position of comprehension (Noddings, 1984). Intersubjectivity occurs in an encounter when each person is able to apprehend the other's subjective world (Parse, 1981; Engel, 1980). There is, in fact, a coming together and a sharing of realities (Mayeroff, 1971). In this sharing, one must be willing to subjectively experience the other's emotions as a basis for understanding.

In copresence, each person in the encounter is fully present and aware of the other as a thinking responding being (Ray, 1981). Riemen (1986) describes being fully present as bringing to a situation one's whole self; the emotional, physical, and cognitive responses to a situation, as well as an awareness of the other not as an object but as another presence with his or her own complex set of responses. In copresence each participant has freedom of choice concerning their involvement in the interaction, and responsibility for the choices made (Paterson & Zderad, 1976).

Taken together, intersubjective copresence means being receptive to the humanity in the other, so that an empathic encounter occurs. One must integrate the logical, empirical, embodied, and creative ways of knowing in order to experience the power of the other's emotions through intuition, precognition, and active transpersonal communication. Traditionally, although it is through the feminine that we experience this type of caring experience, the "masculine" or structural/logical brain is equally important in guiding nursing actions through the myriad of technological, medical, and humanistic interventions needed by clients. Of course, it is by the integration of the various aspects of our beings that enables us to engage in humanistically oriented intersubjective copresence. When intersubjective copresence occurs in a caring interaction, both individuals are aware of sharing a unique experience.

Perception

Perception is each person's unique worldview, which undergoes continuous modification as the person interprets new experiences based on past experiences, values, and knowledge (Horner, 1984; Wood, 1980). A person's perception in any situation guides his or her interpretation of the situation and determines an appropriate behavioral response (Conway, 1978). To comprehend another's perception, one must analyze that perception in a situational context, since perception is different from one context to another (King, 1981).

Again, perception is defined as the individual's dynamic worldview, which is then refined within the situational context, and guides proceeding actions. For caring to take place, the person must be able to perceive the other as a unique being, and interact with the other based on that perception. Perception, however, differs from intersubjective copresence, in that perception may be determined through objective measures, while intersubjective copresence can only be known subjectively (Paterson & Zderad, 1976).

Humanistic Goals

For this model, humanistic goals of caring include client identified goals, the support of development, and health (Leininger, 1981, 1984; Mayeroff, 1971).

Health is both a socially and individually defined state of well being, but it is not the absence of illness. Health includes the ability to function in roles, the continuation of development, and a high state of well being. For example, a well-controlled diabetic could be defined both individually and socially as experiencing health. However, a bipolar depressive in a state of mania would describe him or herself as healthy, but society would not agree with this self-diagnosis.

Watson (1979) discusses the importance of supporting development of the individual and asserts that while most nurses are aware of the biological changes that accompany chronologic development, they must also be attentive to the subtle, inner changes operating psychosocially. Each life phase brings with it particular psychosocial problems that require particular resolutions. Development here includes the physiological and maturational changes of humans as well as the individual's striving to achieve his or her fullest potential, or self-actualization.

ASSUMPTIONS AND PROPOSITIONS

In retrospect, this caring model is based on the following assumptions:

1. The caring person perceives the other's feelings and is responsive to the other as a unique individual (Watson, 1985).
2. The accuracy of perception increases the effectiveness of a person's actions and choices toward attaining humanistic goals (King, 1981).
3. The experience of intersubjective copresence occurs in caring situations, when each person perceives the other as a unique, responsive being.
4. Caring effects, and is effected by, a person's ability to perceive the other's reality.
5. Negative perceptions will decrease caring and reduce the attainability of the humanistic goals.

From these assumptions, the following propositions have been generated:

1. Intersubjective copresence will enhance the perception of the caring.
2. Clarifying a client's perception, through caring, may increase the attainment of humanistic goals.
3. Clarifying the perceptions of nurses and clients may increase instances of experiencing intersubjective copresence in caring.

CONTRIBUTION TO NURSING SCIENCE

Nursing science is the base of knowledge underlying human responses and social interactions in situations of potential or actual health and wellness problems, which can occur across the life span (Gortner, 1980). This model focuses on caring, which by definition as an interpersonal interaction with feeling and behavioral responses has the potential to contribute to nursing science.

While nursing is not clearly defined in the model, caring is an interaction in which a nurse engages. Still, this definition does not equate nursing and caring. Considering the lay population's complaint about the lack of caring, it can not be assumed that all of the behaviors in which a nurse engages are equivalent to caring. Caring is a qualitatively different interaction from the usual tasks and caretaking activities in which most nurses are involved.

This caring model provides an explanation of the interrelationship of the phenomena of caring, perception, intersubjective copresence, and humanistic goals. It also provides a different perspective for viewing these phenomena, and, therefore, contributes to nursing science as it guides an individual's exploration of nurse–client interactions (Meleis, 1987). Because the concepts are defined abstractly and are not culturally delimited, the model's generalizability to many populations increases.

The propositions outlined in the model provide some ideas for testing the model. The propositions also suggest ways of influencing the phenomena, which, if tested, could lead to prediction.

TESTABILITY OF THE MODEL

The proposed model of caring identifies feelings and behaviors as important components of interactions which are directed toward humanistic goals. Because ethnographic methodology focuses on the feelings, thoughts, and

Figure 1
Caring Model Schema

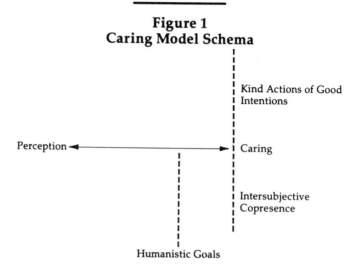

Legend: Solid line indicates continuum of caring from low degree of subjectivity to high degree of subjectivity.
Open lines indicate dynamic exchanges as each component influences the
other.

behaviors of people in their daily lives, with the researcher becoming partially
immersed in the subjects' lived experiences (Leininger, 1985), such methodology might be most appropriate for studying caring. In addition, ethnography is
an appropriate methodology when very little is known about a culture's experience of the phenomena under consideration (Leininger, 1985).

Another qualitative methodology which can be used to study the experience of intersubjective copresence is phenomenology. Phenomenology is used
to explore a phenomenon, categorize it's defining parameters, and suggest
propositions for testing the linkage between the phenomenon and associated
concepts (Meleis, 1987). Phenomenology also appears heuristically valid when
considering the lived caring experience.

Quantitative methodologies are of service here as well. One proposition
pertinent to quantitative analysis pertains to the effect of clarifying perception
on the attainment of humanistic goals. Quantitative tools can measure a client's
perception of experiences and the impact of interventions and interactions over
time on the attainment of humanistic goals. This data then can be subjected to
statistical procedures for enhancement of scope. Comparison between groups
on these measures, or the use of alternative interventions, can be made and
contribute to the body of nursing intervention knowledge.

However, in order to gain a more accurate image of the true complexity of caring interactions, the study of intersubjective copresence should utilize the qualitative methodologies discussed—to explore meanings of the experience for the client. According to Meleis (1987), use of feminist methods such as description, multiple approaches to data gathering, incorporation of the client's perceptions, and the contextuality of the situation can provide for a revision in knowledge development.

These are just a few suggested mechanisms for testing the model presented (see Figure 1). However, when considering this caring model, many different ideas may come to mind. For example, what is the link between this model and nursing practice? Is the value of this model not that it identifies prescription for interventions, but that it supports the nurse's openness with clients, and encourages the sharing of the client's subjective experiences? There is no doubt that caring has the potential for improving client health and supporting individual development. It remains an important phenomena for nursing science.

REFERENCES

Boyle, J. S. (1981). An application of the structural—functional method to the phenomena of caring. In M. M. Leininger (Ed.), *Caring an essential human need* (pp. 37–47). Thorofare, NJ: Slack.

Carper, B. A. (1986). The ethics of caring. In P. L. Chin (Ed.), *Ethical issues in nursing* (pp. 1–9). Rockville, MD: Aspen.

Conway, M. E. (1978). Theoretical approaches to the study of roles. In M. E. Hardy & M. E. Conway (Eds.), *Role theory perspectives for health professionals* (pp. 17–27). New York: Appleton-Century-Crofts.

Engel, N. S. (1980). Confirmation and validation: The caring that is professional nursing. *Image, 12*(3), 53–56.

Gadow, S. A. (1985). Nurse and patient: The caring relationship. In A. H. Bishop & J. R. Scudder (Eds.), *Caring, curing, coping,* (pp. 31–43). Tuscaloosa: The University of Alabama Press.

Gortner, S. R. (1980). Nursing science in transition. *Nursing Research, 29*(3), 180–183. In L. H. Nicoll (Ed.), *Perspectives on nursing theory* (pp. 65–71). Boston: Little, Brown.

Horner, S. D. (1984). *The effect of mothers' participation in a neonatal assessment on their perceptions of their infants.* Unpublished master's thesis, Medical College of Georgia, Augusta, GA.

King, I. M. (1981). *A theory for nursing.* New York: John Wiley and Sons.

Leininger, M. (1981). The phenomena of caring: Importance, research questions and theoretical considerations. In M. Leininger (Ed.), *Caring an essential human need* (pp. 3–15). Thorofare, NJ: Slack.

Leininger, M. (1984). Care: The essence of nursing a health. In M. Leininger (Ed.), *Care the essence of nursing and health* (pp. 3–15). Thorofare, NJ: Slack.

Leininger, M. (1985). Ethnography and ethnonursing: Models and modes of qualitative data analysis. In M. Leininger (Ed.), *Qualitative research methods in nursing* (pp. 33–71). Orlando, Fl.: Grune & Stratton.

Mayeroff, M. (1971). *On caring.* New York: Harper & Row.

McKechnie, J. L. (Ed.). (1983). *Webster's new universal unabridged dictionary.* New York: Simon and Schuster.

Meleis, A. I. (1987). Revisions in knowledge development: A passion for substance. *Scholarly Inquiry for Nursing Practice: An International Journal, 1*(1), 5–19.

Noddings, N. (1984). *Caring, a feminine approach to ethics and moral education.* Berkeley: University of California Press.

Parse, R. R. (1981). Caring from a human science perspective. In M. M. Leininger (Ed.), *Caring an essential human need,* (pp. 129–132). Thorofare, NJ: Slack.

Paterson, J. G., & Zderad, L. T. (1976). *Humanistic nursing.* New York: John Wiley and Sons.

Paulen, A., & Rapp, C. (1981, February). Person-centered caring. *Nursing Management,* 17–21.

Pellegrino, E. D. (1985). The caring ethic: The relation of physician to patient. In A. H. Bishop & J. R. Scudder (Eds.), *Caring, curing, coping* (pp. 8–30). Tuscaloosa: The University of Alabama Press.

Ray, M. A. (1981). A philosophical analysis of caring within nursing. In M. M. Leininger (Ed.), *Caring an essential human need* (pp. 25–36). Thorofare, NJ: Slack.

Reverby, S. (1987). A caring dilemma: Womanhood and nursing in historical perspective. *Nursing Research, 36*(1), 5–11.

Riemen, D. J. (1986). The essential structure of a caring interaction: Doing phenomenology. In P. L. Munhall & C. J. Oiler (Eds.), *Nursing research a qualitative perspective* (pp. 85–108). Norwalk, CT: Appleton-Century-Crofts.

Watson, J. (1979). *Nursing the philosophy and science of caring.* Boston: Little, Brown.

Watson, J. (1985). *Nursing, human science and human care.* Norwalk, CT: Appleton-Century-Crofts.

Wolf, Z. R. (1986). The caring concept and nurse identified caring behaviors. *Topics in Clinical Nursing, 8*(2), 84–93.

Wood, M. J. (1980). Implementing the Riehl interaction model in nursing administration. In Riehl, J. P., & Roy, C. (Eds.), *Conceptual models for nursing practice* (pp. 357–361). Norwalk, CT: Appleton-Century-Crofts.

11

Mental Health:
The Politics of Self-Care

Denise Webster

When I was first asked to write this paper, I proposed that each of the doctoral students involved in the conference at hand write a page about their most personal life concern. I would then string these expressions into a longer paper and hope that this seeming flight of ideas would be of interest to other readers. However, since the students were not as sisterly about my suggestion as I had hoped, I am stuck with publicly displaying my own struggle with the concepts of mental health, politics, nursing, health care delivery, feminism, and related issues. Because this struggle involves as well a severe middle-age crisis in values, the ideas here can seem, at times, to reflect that crisis. An occasional sense of confusion, ambivalence, and, more often, of hypocrisy does appear.

At bottom, I am of at least two minds about everything—which I attribute to having grown up as a woman in a society in which men have provided most prevailing definitions of reality. A common situation for many women, it has resulted in women's experiences either being unnamed or misnamed—although it's equally likely that, for me, my indecisiveness was a result of traumatic toilet training or from being dropped on my head. Because multiple theories to explain any phenomenon always compete for precedence, in choosing which theories to use, which to reject, which to develop in my own work with clients and in teaching, multiple questions arise. As a result, and as a way of avoiding such questions, therapists in all fields try to get away with this simple blind. We describe our interactions with clients as "eclectic therapy"—which is a safe way to say we hope we won't be held to any one position. If we don't or can't attach a clear meaning to our therapy, then we are not obligated to be evaluated on whether we have done what we said we were going to do—always my first choice.

However, I strongly believe that the power to name phenomena is the essence of political power. If I can control the meaning ascribed to something, I can control the situation in which that meaning evolves. And though I usually eschew crude and barbaric concepts such as control, I have experienced, as have most of us, the disturbing effects of having others distort our experiences as they name them. Although many of us are uncomfortable with the concepts of power and control, if we do not actively participate in defining our own reality, then we are abdicating an essential aspect of our search for honesty and integrity in our lives—and we leave open the possibility that others will name our experience to meet their, rather than our, needs.

Since I am of the old "personal is political" school, I offer both personal and social experiences as examples. In the early 1970s, I woke one day to find myself living in a suburb of Chicago, with a different name, with three small children, a husband who traveled most of the time, and a disturbing realization that it had been six years since I had even had time to think of what I had wanted to do with my life. I was certain it wasn't what I was doing—but the process of moving every year, fluctuating hormone levels, and too many years' of exposure to Sesame Street and Mr. Roger's neighborhood had apparently anesthetized my brains enough so that I had no idea where or how to start to think about it. At the urging of a new friend I had met, I made an appointment to see her husband, whom she assured me was a very understanding therapist who had worked with many women. What better referral than from a man's wife? I had never seen a shrink, and I was more than a bit nervous when I went to the first session.

He was, indeed, comforting. As I tried to articulate my feelings and listed my concerns, he nodded sympathetically. When I said I thought that what I really needed was to go back to work—that I had been wanting to do that for years without support from my husband to make it possible—he asked me how I would honestly feel about leaving three small children alone with a stranger during their most important formative years? Vaguely experiencing that representation as guilt provoking, I said I felt ambivalent about that. "Ambivalence," he assured me, was a technical term which was much too complicated for me to truly grasp. What I was, he suggested, was just "confused." He then asked me about the quality of my sex life. I asked him what that had to do with my wanting to go back to work. He sighed, shook his head with pity and said, "Well, in my experience, women who want to leave the home, aren't getting what they need—so to speak—at home," as he reached over and put his hand on my knee. This, I later learned, was the exact definition of women's mental health problems which he had given to many of his female clients. Apparently, there was an epidemic of this diagnostic problem among the clients in his practice. When I did not return to any sessions with him, his wife reported to me sadly that he saw me as having a problem with trust, and he hoped I would get the help I so badly needed.

My point is to remind us that the concept of caring raises numerous feelings of ambivalence in women. Ambivalence also has many meanings and if we're not clear about those meanings for ourselves, we may not only end up getting screwed, but also paying for the presumed pleasure.

I think this situation is a just one example of the confusion many women feel in trying to balance or prioritize their need to care for others and their need to care for themselves—a phenomenon often called "selfishness" when observed in women. Often, an additional confusion arises between this personal ambivalence and the social demand that women feel and act caring (particularly to men, children, and aging in-laws) since it is both our "duty" and our natural "inclination." It is with this issue that I am probably most hypocritical. And I always far prefer pointing out other's hypocrisies than in finding myself, enduring my own.

Often, I place one foot on the bandwagon that proclaims that women are just more capable of being nurturing, more sensitive to other's needs, more able to stay and work on difficult relationships. These are all qualities I value highly. I also want to believe that people can change, that through socialization or teaching, people (i.e., men) can learn to be nurturing and caring. I believe that fathers should be very involved in the care and nurture of their children— that is, if they are going to care for them in ways that I see as caring and nurture those values that I see as important. If they are merely going to nurture principally male ideas about status and power and winning, then that's another story. If we're going to socialize a son with different values than those just mentioned, then that son must be protected from a kind of fatherly advice that supports the presumed pleasures of gaining status and power over others.

I enthusiastically join in doctor-bashing too. I commiserate with others and add my own stories about despicable physicians who don't evaluate anything beyond physical signs, who think that dramatic chemical or surgical intervention is the only answer to health problems. Clearly these poor misinformed creatures should not be permitted to practice without the healthy balance of a nurse. I also know that when I've been sick for any length of time I want my doctor to make me well immediately. And then I bristle with irritation when I hear physicians say that they are holistic—that they spend time with patients getting to know them, that they consider alternative therapies, and look at lifestyle in working with patients. That's why they don't need to have other health care personnel in their offices. Maybe that's why they think they can develop a new category of worker—the Registered Care Technologist (RCT)— since they themselves will now be providing the coordination and broad overview of the client's needs. "How dare they encroach on our territory?" I rant.

I should probably be more embarrassed to describe my own conflictive thoughts about these issues, but since former President Reagan was recently discovered to be open to alternative ways of knowing, I feel confident that readers will excuse my ambivalence once they know I'm a Libra—I can't help weighing all sides of all issues. Perhaps I'm the only one who does this, but I don't think so.

When my mother was dying and had just gone into a deep coma, my father (who was not a Libra) remarked, "Well, I think she's going to be OK, don't you?" I was speechless. He then immediately asked if I would mind accompanying him. I asked where and he said "to buy a cemetery plot." In working with cancer patients and their families, we have come to see such normal "craziness" as expected behavior for those on a roller coaster between the highs and lows of hope and despair—a pattern quite typical in nurses too. We hope for the best and prepare for the worst. But as we shuttle between both positions we look to others, and feel ourselves a little "crazy" in the bargain.

What does this have to do with *self-care* or *caring* and what we call things? I am well aware that the major theories about self-care and caring have similar components. In their totality, both address the perspective of those receiving care and those giving care. But in the emphasis each places on one aspect or the other, less immediately apparent implications arise. Again, it boils down to what you call something, how you define it—which concepts are presented as central versus those which are addressed only in the process of fleshing out the theory as a whole.

In this light, and taken in their extremes, it might be argued that the self-care theory is probably consistent with the realist in us. It may also express covertly or overtly an intensely male perspective on how things should be done.

Originally, I was attracted to the concept of self-care because I believed in its emphasis—as I perceived it—on the patient's right to self-determination about health care. This acknowledgement that we take care of ourselves most of the time and in understanding our experiences, understand best what works and does not work for us, was salutory. It provided a fine balance to the overbearing arrogant decision making by so-called experts who used professional distance and mystification of health care to terrorize their sick patients into compliance with health plans that had been given to them without consideration of their perceptions of their own needs. If you were involved in the women's health movement in the late 1960s or early 1970s, such rhetoric might sound familiar. Self-care, with it's emphasis on the professional's supplying only those compensatory actions which the client cannot provide for herself, was a distinct improvement in balancing the power between professionals and patients.

The term *self-care* had then, as now, numerous meanings—from the women's health movement emphasis on knowing one's body and doing self-inspection of cervical changes across menstrual cycles, to the view in alternative medicine that people could carry out technical procedures for themselves if they had the right equipment and books to explain the procedures. At the social level, self-care included concepts of self-help and mutual aid, and encouraged the development of self-help groups organized around particular conditions. It broke down the isolation of the individual and helped people to learn different ways of coping from each other. They could even teach each other about the condition and about how to demand from physicians and others the treatment that was most appropriate, based on current information to which lay people now had increased access.

This focus on actions which can be taught to patients is consistent in the nursing literature on self-care. Orem's (1985) concept makes it clear that care is multidimensional, but that nursing is concerned with deliberate actions which can be learned. Identification of self-care needs and the processes or technologies to meet those needs are described among the basic propositions. The presuppositions include that "all things being equal, human beings have the potential to develop their intellectual and practical skills and the motivation essential for self-care and care of dependent family members." What happens when all things aren't equal is not so clear. Pender's (1987) book on self-care addresses the topic similarly, saying that self-care is a major theme in current health care policy. Pender's book focused thereafter on how nurses could help clients develop competence for self-care. Pender defines self-care as an ongoing activity as well as a competence to be developed through self-care plans and programs for health promotion.

So far, so good. As a philosophy of care, self-care has significant appeal. It is, in fact, peculiarly American in it's tendency to value independence, assertiveness, self-competence, and action in the individual who is in need of health care services. It also has a familiar feel to it, which I was finally able to identify when I read the two quotes that preface the book edited by Riehl-Sisca (1985), *The Science and Art of Self-Care*. The first quote is by Ralph

Waldo Emerson: "Our chief want in life is somebody who shall make us do what we can." It leaves little doubt that the goal of such an approach is self-sufficiency. The second quote was even more familiar, Rudyard Kipling's "Someday you will be a man, my son."

For those of you who were not raised with Rudyard Kipling, you have a treat in store. I was ruminating about this poem which had dominated my entire childhood, when I found that it is widely used in those nauseatingly insipid cards that one can buy now—the kind that shows sunsets and has odes to someone's pearly teeth, and equally saccharine sentiments. Kipling would probably not have approved of any of these cards, including the one his poem is on, a birthday card entitled "*IF*" *FOR BOYS*.

> *If you can keep your head when all about you are losing theirs, and*
> *blaming it on you,*
> *If you can trust yourself when all men doubt you, but make al-*
> *lowance for their doubting too;*
> *If you can wait and not be tired by waiting, or being lied about, don't*
> *deal in lies,*
> *Or being hated, don't give way to hating,*
> *And yet don't look too good nor talk too wise;*
> *If you can dream and not make dreams your master, if you can*
> *think and not make dreams your aim,*
> *If you can meet with triumph and disaster, and treat those two*
> *imposters just the same;*
> *If you can bear to hear the truth you've spoken twisted by knaves to*
> *make a trap for fools,*
> *Or watch the things you gave your life to, broken,*
> *And stoop and build'em up with worn-out tools;*
>
> *If you can make one heap of all your winnings,*
> *And risk it on one turn of pitch-and-toss,*
> *And lose, and start again at your beginnings,*
> *And never breathe a word about your loss;*
>
> *If you can force your heart and nerve and sinew*
> *To serve your turn long after they are gone,*
> *And so hold on when there is nothing in you*
> *Except the will which says to them:"Hold on!"*
>
> *If you can talk with crowds and keep your virtue,*
> *Or walk with kings —nor lose the common touch,*
> *If neither foes nor loving friends can hurt you,*
> *If all men count with you, but none too much;*

If you can fill the unforgiving minute
with sixty seconds worth of distance run,
Yours is the Earth and everything that's in it,
And —which is more —you'll be a man, my Son!

It brings tears to my eyes—and makes the hair stand up on the back of my neck—when I think about this for any length of time. Here are all those fine male values we know and love, perhaps best captured in the series of "RAMBO" films starring Sylvester Stallone—macho men, who remain, somehow above it all, noble in their lonely struggle and untouched by emotion, unemcumbered by any concern with others' needs. And yet it still has a certain appeal, doesn't it? Preserving a patient's dignity and independence are central nursing values and it certainly captures those qualities.

However, the potential limitations to this kind of value system are beginning to appear (too clearly!) in the current health care system. Gartner and Riessman (1977) wrote more than a decade ago—speaking specifically of the self-help movement—that despite the positive aspects of self-care and self-help, there are also potential dangers, which are likely to become apparent in a climate of scarcity and economizing. While the intention was that self-help service supplement existing service, it may come to pass that the self-help approach is increasingly proposed as an alternative to the needed human services. Certainly it is cheaper and reduces the strain on the existing system. It may also result in volunteers (or family members who have to carry out care) being pitted against employed workers and competing when it is cooperation that is greatly needed.

Another possibility Gartner and Riessman foresaw was victim blaming, which can divert attention from the responsibilities of the system and professionals. Ultimately this can result in a diminution of existing services which are not actually replaced by the self-care efforts. This approach, they point out, has always been used with poor and minority groups, who are encouraged to pull themselves up by their bootstraps, rather than demanding better economic opportunities. The dilemma is that services might not be provided at all unless alternative or self-help approaches exist. Yet the presence of such approaches permits the system to ignore the changes it might otherwise be forced to incorporate.

Furthermore, as Gartner and Riessman point out, an overemphasis on the self, rather than on the social structure can lead to escapism, narcissism, and privatism. The emphasis on the individual and client-centered approaches may diminish the attention to the larger social system and structural changes that are necessary to deal with larger social problems.

How important are these concerns 10 years later? Certainly in the area of mental health and women's mental health there has been a long history of blaming the victim—in theories that held women responsible for not only their own problems but those of husbands and children. Currently, the chronically mentally ill are classified as a major social problem—one that is seen as insurmountable without great expense to society. Furthermore, the emphasis on independence, self-determination, and personal responsibility is a source of continual conflict in situations in which the very lack of ability to take personal responsibility may be among the major mental health problems a client exhibits.

As helpful as self-care theories such as Orem's (1985) are, they have not been particularly useful in addressing larger social systems or circumstances in which the client is unable to provide adequate self-care. Nor is it clearly a situation requiring partial or whole compensation—that is, it usually seems that the client is simply lacking in necessary motivation to care for him or her self.

The concept of responsibility for the problem and responsibility for the solution in health care situations has been addressed by Brickman et al. (1982) in their work on models of helping and coping. The very popularity of concepts such as stress and coping should alert us to the implication that help is something given to people who are either not seen as responsible for the problem or the solution—as in the medical model. When people are perhaps held responsible for the problem and probably for the solution, then the concept of coping becomes more salient. However, there is always the potential with this kind of self-care model that the focus on the individual's rights and responsibilities will be used to justify abandonment by professionals of undesirable tasks and undesirable people in the name of protecting the individual's freedom of choice. Clearly this is only one horn of the dilemma.

The ideal of autonomy and independence has usually been most highly valued and promulgated by men like Kipling as he appears in the poem. To be a woman in a society in which men value independence and autonomy for themselves and something perhaps different for women is also destined to lead to some ambivalence about dependence and independence in women. Doing a series of literature reviews on women and mental health has helped me to see the patterns emerging in books that purport to address women's health concerns. Particularly in popular literature, there is a move from anger and separatism, to making it in a man's world, to concern about our biologic clocks and, more recently, to concern about how to catch, maintain and change the "man of your choice." From this vantage, it's difficult to know if we are seeing a predictable swing of the pendulum that will eventually balance, or if we're witnessing a loss of ground and cooptive renaming of what the women's movement is about (Webster, 1988). No wonder we're confused.

Mitchell and Oakley (1986) point out that "women's right to enter a man's world" is both demanded and criticized. The ambivalence which the issue arouses is important because it indicates areas of uncertainty and confusion about feminist aims, a confusion which might be more productive than a "premature clarity." This comes as a relief. I now can reframe my ambivalence as healthy open-mindedness.

Our ambivalence about caring is parallelled by our ambivalence about motherhood, as both Addriene Rich (1986) and Angela McBride (1973) have pointed out. Women often feel confused between the socially demanded institution of motherhood and the personal experience of motherhood, which is distorted by institutional demands (Mitchell & Oakley, 1986).

In case you should doubt that socialization for women—caring for and oriented toward others' needs—is still with us, I offer the following evidence. When I gave a version of this paper for the original presentation, I quoted a poem, "IF for Girls," by Gale Baker Stanton, I found on a greeting card. Based on the same structure and presentation of "ideals" that Kipling used in the original poem, this card presented a picture of a "successfully grown" girl-into-woman. Several women have reported that they recall being given the same card at important transition points, such as graduations or birthdays. The essence of the poem was that a "real woman" would be recognized by her ability to be self-effacing, to be generous toward others, to contribute to maintenance of the social fabric, and to value her special gifts, her strength, and her abilities in terms of their potential benefit for others. It is, in its own way, a very moving poem. My point had been to demonstrate the sharp contrast posed by the juxtaposition of the two poems. I have sometimes made the same point to undergraduate students by playing the 1945 "Soliloquy" from the Rodgers and Hammerstein musical "Carousel." Usually students assure me that times have changed, that nobody gets those messages these days, and that maybe (even though I am going to give them a grade in this class) I am making mountains out of mole hills. Maybe they are right. But when we tried to obtain permission to reprint the poem mentioned above (along with other sections of poetry and prose used as examples herein) permission was denied by the publisher. They disapproved, we were told, of the context in which it was being presented. If it were being put into a religiously-oriented collection, or some publication that did not question the desirability of the sentiments expressed, such permissions would have been granted. The appropriate socialization of women, therefore, will not be demolished in this publication. At least not verbatim.

Altruism was much more clearly expected of the person receiving this card—in fact it would seem that the essence of what she is to be valued for is her capacity to meet the needs of those around her—which brings me to the topic of caring. I am one of those diploma nurses who came into nursing in answer to a calling—unfashionable these days, but there it is. I won't embarrass people here by taking a vote on this issue, but more than half of the nurses I interviewed while doing my master's thesis also had the same experience and claim, as many do now, that nursing just feels "right" to them. It is the caring component which is most attractive in this group and presumably to many here. Since much of this conference has focused on caring I won't belabor the point, but I contend that, again although in total it may contain many of the elements addressed in theories of self-care, in caring theories much of the focus is on the emotions, affect, or behavior of the provider of care. In defense of the other view, it must be acknowledged that Gaut (in Watson) makes the point that caring must always be manifested in concrete acts, and that caring actions must be judged solely on the welfare of the person being cared for. Watson (1985) and Mayeroff (1971) also address the needs of the caregiver, and importance of caring for the self as for another. The concept of growth of personhood for the nurse and patient through practice of caring is clearly stated. However, the major emphasis remains on the thoughts, feelings, and behavior of the carer as opposed to the emphasis on the required actions of the patient, as in self-care. Certainly both sides of the equation are represented when one takes both theories into consideration.

For example, Watson's (1985) carative factors address first a humanist-altruistic system of values, and stress the need for compassion and empathy as the contexts for the caring experience. Since I have mellowed as I have gotten older, and also feel less confident that I will be able to provide my own self-care completely, I am now attracted to the idea that the focus should be on caring, rather than self-care if a choice must be made.

Perhaps.

Although I like this idea, I also sometimes feel the burden of caring as a palpable creeping exhaustion under too many demands. I really do believe, as I wrote in a chapter about the oppression of women, that

> While the ability to nurture others is perhaps a woman's most powerful strategy to control others (and the sine-qua-non of valued stereotypic female characteristics), it is also the potential source of her despair. Nurturing, to the extent that it is required of women, is perhaps the essence of oppression within the female experience. It is demanded, but must be given freely. It is not necessarily expected to be reciprocated in kind. (Webster, 1986)

The demand to do something spontaneously is the hallmark of the paradoxical double bind—and thus our ambivalence, or at least mine. I would like to be caring, but resent heartily the expectation that I must care. (Reverby, 1987, has addressed this paradox in her book Ordered to Care.)

There is much to find attractive in models which are organized around caring, but we must remember here, too, the capacity for our strengths to be used against us. Self-sacrifice is highly suspect in a society which values the individual and the illusion of independence above all other values.

In fact, it is so suspect that there is now a DSMIII-R experimental category which makes self-sacrifice a diagnostic category of personality disorder. Actually if one reads closely, it seems that it's not so much the sacrifice as it is complaining about the sacrifice that will get one labelled as having Self-Defeating Personality Disorder. If one sacrifices silently, or is truly altruistic and doesn't point out the sacrifice, the label isn't applicable. But I'm not sure Mother Theresa would escape this classification. According to the American Psychiatric Association (1987), the criteria for this category include the following (my interpolations are bracketed):

A. *A pervasive pattern of self-defeating behavior, beginning by early adulthood and present in a variety of contexts. The person may often avoid or undermine pleasurable experiences, be drawn to situations or relationships in which he or she will suffer, and prevent others from helping him or her, as indicated by a least five of the following:*

1. chooses people and situations that lead to disappointment, failure, or mistreatment even when better options are clearly available. [Clear to the person making the diagnosis.]

2. rejects or renders ineffective the attempts of others to help him or her [i.e. tries to retain independence].

3. following positive personal events (e.g. new achievement), responds with depression, guilt or a behavior that produces pain (e.g. an accident). [All analysts know there is no such thing as an "accident".]

4. incites angry or rejecting responses from others and then feels hurt, defeated, or humiliated (e.g. makes fun of spouse in public, provoking an angry retort, then feels devastated). [I wonder who wrote this one?]

5. rejects opportunities for pleasure, or is reluctant to acknowledge enjoying himself or herself (despite having adequate social skills and the capacity for pleasure) [i.e. has learned that making any personal plans will cause children to come down with chicken pox].

6. fails to accomplish tasks crucial to his or her personal objectives despite demonstrated ability to do so (e.g. helps fellow students write papers, but is unable to write his or her own). [This person would qualify for mother of the year, however, for making a halloween costume on the only day available to finish a midterm project.]

7. is uninterested in or rejects people who consistently treat him or her well (e.g. is unattracted to caring sexual partners). [for example, a caring therapist?]

8. engages in excessive self-sacrifice that is unsolicited by the intended recipients of the sacrifice. [Good mothers anticipate needs — and it's so tacky to have to ask someone to do your laundry and fix your meals.]

B. *The behaviors in A do not occur exclusively in response to, or in anticipation of, being physically, sexually, or psychologically abused. [There is evidence that any of the foregoing may result in a form of brainwashing in which the person is either unaware of being psychologically abused or feels the treatment is justified — i.e. by definition this person is unlikely to report this exclusionary information.]*

C. *The behaviors in A do not occur only when the person is depressed [i.e. most women probably will be ineligible for the label anyway at the current rate of depression among women].*

Two students in the graduate psychiatric nursing program, Sue Orahood and Bari Platter (1988), recently wrote an interesting paper which points out that nurses, working in underpaid, overworked situations with rotating shifts and holidays spent on the job—often working double shifts to cover for the shortage of staff in the area and often feeling unappreciated—are, by definition, suffering from this personality disorder. I have often thought that one way to supplement nurses' salaries would be to give them all an automatic diagnosis of self-defeating personality disorder, do a mass blessing or therapy session at weekly intervals, and give them all third party payment reimbursement in recognition of their mental distress as an added pay incentive to continue their disturbed behavior.

Obviously we know that nurses aren't just self-sacrificing or even always caring. The existing public images of nurses often reflect the tendency to see things in polarities or dichotomies—and may also account for much of the ambivalence I have been describing. Nurses are portrayed as either sweet and dumb, possibly sexy, and maybe masochistic or as cold-hard top-sergeants forcing patients to do things to become independent in ways which reveal the nurses' underlying sadism. The ethic for firm and kind care that most of us were given gets lost in the tendency to be able to hold only one image at a time. The problem is intensified by our lack of a language that can embrace two opposing thoughts at the same time unless we create oxymorons—such as the concept of *Tough Love*, or, as in Adrienne Rich's (1979) poem, which starts out "A wild patience has taken me this far."

Interestingly, a study of thinking styles, as reported in a book by Harrison and Bramson (1982), described a particular split kind of thinking as being quite typical of nurses. They identified five general styles of thinking held by what they labelled "pragmatists," "synthesists," "analysts," "idealists," and "realists." While many people have one predominant style of thinking, many others have two. Among the more illogical combinations is the realist-idealist. Although there are few examples of thinking styles associated with particular professions, this was specifically illustrated by discussing nurses, which I find fascinating. They describe idealists as follows:

> *Idealists look and respond attentively and receptively. They show a supportive, open smile. They do a good deal of head-nodding. They give verbal and nonverbal feedback that serves to encourage you to be open with them, to trust them, to see them as helpful and receptive. They may not be aggressive in offering their own ideas and opinions, but they listen and they welcome yours.*
>
> *Idealists are apt to express their feelings, their values, their ideas about what is good for people, the community, society. They express concern about goals and the long-range aspects of things.*
>
> *The tone of Idealists tends to be hopeful and inquiring. They ask a lot of questions, but sometimes their questions sound tentative, even apologetic. They don't like to step on other people's toes, or to sound challenging. Above all, they are uncomfortable with conflict or open argument. They want people to agree, and to be "nice" to each other, and they often will show, in their openness and receptivity, a strong tendency to trust others, sometimes more than is wise.*
>
> *Idealists enjoy feeling-level discussion about people and their problems, and abstract discussions about philosophy and ethics—so long as the discussion does not become acrimonious. They dislike talk that seem data-bound, too heavily factual, or "dehumanizing." They hate openly conflictual argument.* (p. 29)

The Idealist grand strategy is labelled assimilative thinking and is based on two basic Idealist assumptions:

> *The first assumption is that the world can be a better place, and people can live together in it harmoniously, if only they can agree on overall goals. That is, the Idealist believes that disagreement and differences can be assimilated and harmonized.*
>
> *The second is what we might call the "holistic" assumption. Everything is connected with everything else. In order to understand any*

problem, we need to look at the total context. It is another form of assimilation, in which we try to look at the relationships of things and events with a broad perspective. (pp. 31–32)

The Realist they describe as follows:

Realists tend to have a direct, forceful, frank appearance —not necessarily aggressive, but sometimes that too. They are likely to look you smartly in the eye. They express agreement or disagreement quickly, both verbally and nonverbally. In other words, you usually have a pretty good idea of where you stand with a Realist. Some favorite Realist expression are: "it's obvious to me. . ." "Everybody knows that. . ." "Let's look at the facts in the situation. . ."

Realists are quick to express their opinions, and they are more apt than the rest of us to "own" them. That is, they stay away from "weasel words," such as "don't you think. . ." or "Wouldn't you agree that. . .?" They describe things factually. In order to clarify their meanings they give specific examples, or offer short, pointed, descriptive anecdotes.

Realists are apt to be forthright and positive. At times they may sound dogmatic or domineering, especially if your view of the facts is different from theirs.

Realists enjoy direct, factual discussion of immediate matters, the more practical and down-to-earth the better. They use succinct, pithy, descriptive statements. They dislike talk that seems too theoretical, sentimental, subjective, impractical, or long-winded. They like things short, sweet, and concise. Subtlety is not their strong suit. They can't stand "shaggy dog" stories, but they may like puns and plays on words if they are quickly understandable and have punch. They are often hearty, explosive laughers and the humor they like best is likely to be down-to earth, if not earthy. (pp. 68–69)

The Realist grand strategy is based on Empirical Discovery. For them:

What is real in the world is what can be seen, heard, felt, or experienced concretely. The reality of a "fact" is the basic building block of knowledge and understanding of the Realist. Reality cannot be deduced by working from a theory or an abstraction. Reality is INDUCED from observation and experience of facts. That is the empirical approach. . . . (pp. 68–69)

While there are some places where it might seem possible for one person to hold both of these thinking styles, it also is rather suggestive of a dissociative personality to consider what it would be like to have both styles. We may be able to increase our income from third party payments to nurses, if Harrison and Bramson are correct. When describing the Idealist-Realist (IR) combination, Harrison and Bramson say:

> This combination is characterized by a twin thrust of high standards an "concreteness." The IR knows how things "should" be and has at hand practical steps for reaching the "should." A person with the IR combination may often be seen by others as both receptive and immediately helpful. The IR is likely to show considerable drive toward getting things done and achieving high quality results at the same time.

They go on:

> Nurses often tend to show high preferences for both Idealist and Realist strategies. Consider especially the nature of hospital nursing. Think about the motivations that a person must have if he or she is going to be an effective nurse, one who is satisfied with the job.
>
> Nursing requires a commitment to community and personal service, to supportiveness and helpfulness. This is the Idealist part of nursing. Idealists get their rewards from being helpful, and from the internal satisfactions of the work itself and what they see as its high value. Idealists are often content to be unsung heroes. [Which works out nicely].
>
> The Realist part of the combination in nurses is found on the practical, concrete, and immediate aspects of the work. There are specific individuals to be cared for, immediate needs to be met. Every act of hospital nursing achieves a concrete result. There is a dressing to be changed, a shot to be administered, a body to be bathed, a patient to be made more comfortable. There is nothing obscure or ambiguous about the act of nursing, and that appeals strongly to the Realist. (pp. 84–85)

Among the disadvantages of Idealist thinking they include a tendency to be:

> more prone than others to experience dilemmas—often finding themselves in situations where either of two choices is equally unsatisfactory—always wanting to do what is right They may also be very self-effacing and rather than show any resentment or disappointment, resist going against a group position.
>
> The most serious Idealist liability derives from their Idealist great strength—reliance on high standards— . . . sometimes the Idealist'

*standards are set so high that they themselves can't live up to them,
not to mention other people. So Idealists tend to suffer two related
pangs —guilt over disappointment in themselves, and hurt feelings
over disappointment in others. (pp. 41–42) [With luck we'll get a
third diagnosis of Dysphoric Disorder.]*

On the other hand, the disadvantages for the Realist are associated with
being seen as pushy—pushing others to be specific and to take responsibility.
Shades of self-care?
They write:

*Because Realists are people of strong opinions, based on perceived
facts, they are quick to form opinions of other people. Like all of us,
they respect people much like themselves. If you don't stand up to a
Realist, he or she is likely to not respect you. . . . Also . . . they
are sometimes experienced as being stubborn. (pp. 76–77)*

Not surprisingly, then, the Idealist-Realist combination is seen as:

*often having the problem of finding themselves overcommitted
. . . especially to the needs and wants of others. They tend to take
on the burdens of others and not to pay enough attention to themselves. And if those they help don't acknowledge the service, IR's feel
resentful and ill-used. (p. 85)*

There it is—by virtue of our personalities we become nurses and by virtue
of acting out our personalities in nursing we are all suffering from Self-
Defeating Personality Disorder.
Nurses are certainly not unusual in their combining realistic and idealist
ways of thinking. At this point, I will take a leap and claim that Idealism most
closely reflects the stereotypic female caring ethic with the focus on feeling
and welfare of others, while Realism may more accurately reflect a self-care
perspective valuing activity, personal responsibility (often for others), and
independence—predominantly male values.
I also think nurses are not unlike most women in having both sets of values
and being unclear sometimes about what one is doing for oneself versus
for others. Many of the psychological theories stressing the importance of
boundaries tell us that being able to be clear about such things is the essence
of mental health. Not everyone is so sure. At the Stone Center at Wellesley,
research and clinical work with women is helping us to develop a psychology
of women, based on women values and women's experiences. The concepts of

autonomy and independence as evidencing the highest level of maturity are questioned in this model, which is helping us to rename women's experiences using women's own voices. What may eventually come of this and other related work is a better understanding of human experience and a language which helps us to name our realities in ways which don't feel degrading or confusing to us. For now, the language is sparse. One of the best examples is the renaming of passive dependence (when viewed from a different value orientation) to "active connection" (Miller, 1986). This kind of oxymoron as a way of describing what feels to us like self-contradictory polarities may be cumbersome, but it is still an improvement over what we may experience as demeaning, pathologizing, or confusing-making when others name our realities from their own world views.

As a child I had the advantage or disadvantage of being socialized by both parents—parents with highly polarized views of appropriate sex roles. Because of my father's influence I was inclined to engage in activities usually limited to boys and was often called a "tomboy." However, as I grew and began to exhibit the behaviors of my female peers along with "tomboy" behaviors, my mother used to warn me menacingly that the world was not ready for "Hermaphroditic creatures." Psychological testing later also showed these tendencies to be both very feminine and very masculine. This was always presented to me as a problem—one that would probably ruin any chances I had of being a happily adjusted woman. They were right. However, in the interim there is a new word for this constellation of characteristics. *Androgyny* has come to represent a psychological profile which encompasses the conscious use of masculine and feminine characteristics dependent on the context of a situation (Cook, 1986). It is not (at least now) a stigmatizing word, and it is unusual in its ability to encompass the polarities of masculinity and femininity as they are currently constructed.

What I hope for, for nursing, and for our mental health, is that we can name our own experiences and be actively involved in creating and communicating our own definitions of our values of caring and self-care. If we don't, then we will at best be characterized by one of the two polarities. At worst, we may experience a situation in which we are defined as being at least naive idealists, and perhaps as having self-defeating personality disorders. At the same time, we may find ourselves participating passively in the social and institutional abandonment of those who are unable to care for themselves, as well as contributing to the added burden of women to provide needed but unacknowledged and nonreimbursed services to others—which will reinforce the diagnosis of their personal pathology.

It is my hope, as an every-other-day idealist, that we can develop a language which reveals our valuing of ourselves and others. This language must also reveal that the work we do goes beyond just the individual and interpersonal levels to encompass a social sense of caring and responsibility for others with the desire to preserve their dignity and respect their choices.

Sheryl Ruzek (1986), in *Feminist Visions of Health*, warns us that:

> *as self-help, self-care, and social support are increasingly recognized as valuable to the maintenance of health, feminists are concerned that these aspects of the traditional female role will be expected of them either without compensation in the home, or in the form of low-paid paraprofessional work in the formal health care system. [As Registered Care Technologists?] Thus, sharing and caring carry with them the possibility of more humanistic approaches to health care, but also the possibility of women's strengths being used against them.* (p.190)

This is the challenge—to integrate the values of both caring and self-care in ways which are clear enough to us and others so that they defy distortion and eventual use as weapons against us. I hope we can continue to deal with these issues and face this challenge in our everyday work and in future conferences.

REFERENCES

American Psychiatric Association. (1987). *Diagnostic and statistical manual of mental disorders,* (3rd ed. rev). Washington, DC: American Psychiatric Association, pp. 371-374.

Benton, D. W. (1978). *Preprofessional socialization experiences of masters' prepared psychiatric nurses in independent and nonindependent roles.* Unpublished thesis, University of Illinois at the Medical Center, Chicago.

Brickman, P., Rabinowitz, V., Karuza, J., Coates, D., Cohn, E., & Kidder, L. (1982). Models of helping and coping. *American Psychologist 37*(4), 368-384.

Cook, E. (1986). *Psychological androgyny.* New York: Pergamon Press.

Eichenbaum, L., & Orbach, S. (1982). *Understanding women: A feminist psychoanalytic approach.* New York: Basic Books.

Gartner, S., & Reissman, F. (1977). *Self-help in the human services.* San Francisco: Josey-Bass, pp. 119-121.

Harrison, A., & Bramson, R. (1982). *Styles of thinking.* New York: Doubleday, pp. 29, 31-32, 41-42, 68-69, 76-77, 84-85, 85.

Kipling, R. (1990). If. In L. Phillips (Ed.), *The Random House treasury of best-loved poems.* New York: Random House, pp. 173-175.

McBride, A. (1973). *The growth and development of mothers.* New York: Harper & Row.

Mayeroff, M. (1971). *On caring.* New York: Harper & Row.

Miller, J. B. (1986). *Toward a new psychology of women* (2nd ed.). Boston: Beacon Press.

Mitchell, J. & Oakley, A. (1986). *What is feminism: A reexamination.* New York: Pantheon, pp. 127–150.

Orahood, S., & Platter, B. (1988). *Health policy: Self-defeating personality disorder.* Unpublished manuscript. University of Colorado, School of Nursing.

Orem, D. (1985). *Nursing: Concepts of practice.* (3rd ed.) New York: McGraw-Hill.

Pender, N. (1987). *Health promotion in nursing practice* (2nd ed.). Norwalk, CT: Appleton & Lange, p. 185.

Reverby, S. (1987). *Ordered to care: The dilemma of American Nursing, 1850–1945.* New York: Cambridge University Press.

Rich, A. (1979). *A wild patience has taken me this far.* New York: Norton.

Riehl-Sisca, J. (Ed.). (1985). *The science and art of self-care.* Norwalk, CT: Appleton-Century-Crofts.

Rodgers, R., & Hammerstein, O. (1945). "Soliloquy". Copyright 1945 by Williamson Music, Inc., New York, NY. Sole selling agent, T. B. Harms Company.

Ruzek, S. (1986). Feminist visions of health: An international perspective. In J. Mitchell & A. Oakley (Eds.), *What is feminism: A reexamination.* New York: Pantheon, p. 190.

Watson, J. (1985). *Nursing: Human science and human care —a theory of nursing.* Norwalk, CT: Appleton-Century-Crofts, pp. 32, 75.

Webster, D. (1988). Women and mental health. In C. Leppa & C. Miller (Eds.), *Annual Review of women's health.* Phoenix: Oryx Press, pp. 14–33.

Webster, D. (1986). The oppressed client. In J. Durham & S. Hardin (Eds.), *The nurse psychotherapist in private practice.* New York: Springer, pp. 117–130.

12

Mother-Blaming in the Nursing Care of the Chronically Mentally Ill: The Politics of Caregiving

Carol Roberts

Working with the chronically mentally ill as a formal caregiver can be a challenge with few rewards. But what is it like to be the mother of an individual suffering from chronic mental illness? What is it like to have the experience of discovering that one's child is chronically mentally ill? What is it like for the mother, the informal caregiver, as this illness unfolds? What have mothers experienced in interactions with mental health professionals? What are the attitudes of nurses toward these mothers? Do mothers perceive nurses as responsive to their needs?

Review of relevant literature should reflect to what degree these questions have been answered. This review should also identify whether nurses are aware of the experiences of mothers and how responsive nurses are in meeting their needs.

First, however, there is value in situating these questions within an historical and cultural context. There are dynamics that obstruct nurses understanding the experiences of mothers. Historically, mothers have been blamed for causing the mental illnesses of their children. Nurses, as members of an oppressed professional group, may collude with such mother-blaming. Indeed, nurses who behave as members of an oppressed group may be incapable of developing an accurate understanding of the experiences of the mothers of concern. As a result, it is a feminist perspective that motivates me to examine these dynamics and to explore the literature so that nurses can better understand the experiences of mothers involved in caregiving.

Estimates of the number of individuals who are chronically mentally ill in this country range from 1.7–2.5 million. Most of these individuals suffer from schizophrenia, a disease that usually strikes in late adolescence, which developmentally is a time of emancipation from dependence on one's parents. A schizophrenic has disintegrative experiences that alter his or her thoughts, feelings, and perceptions while undermining motivation. This impairment in functioning often prevents the individual from performing the adult tasks of pursuing a career and forming intimate relationships.

Historically, an individual suffering from schizophrenia would have lived his or her life within an institution. In the 1950s, the discovery of medications and the development of social programs provided hope for short hospitalizations and an early return to community living.

Now, decades after efforts to move the mentally ill out of institutions, a financially inadequate, poorly coordinated system exists. The failed goals of the community mental health movement have placed a heavy caregiving burden on family members.

Approximately one half of the chronically mentally ill currently living outside of institutions live with their families. Many others, due to the nature of their illness and the inadequacy of the mental health system, live in the streets. Both living situations leave family members feeling helpless and often frightened.

As stated, in this paper my focus concerns mothers within families where chronic mental illness exists. My reasons for such specificity are multifold. I have worked in mental health settings with the chronically mentally ill for 14 years. I had certainly observed mother-blaming among staff in clinical settings and, in fact, had been guilty of it in my first years of working in mental health nursing. I recently entered the academic setting and found that undergraduate nursing students came to the classroom with the belief that early developmental interactions between the child and mother caused schizophrenia. These assumptions were reinforced with the neutral presentation of theories of schizophrenia in the classroom, theories that I had assumed were outdated. I am also interested in this particular focus because mothers are considered the caregivers of their children; and, as part of this responsibility, they, more than others, have been blamed for what befalls their offspring. Although the experiences of other family members are significant in and of themselves, their experiences still fall outside the parameters of this paper.

Caplan and Hall-McCorquodale (1985) state "since early in this century, mental health professionals have legitimized the tendency of both lay people and professionals to blame mothers for whatever goes wrong with their offspring" (p. 345). Caplan and Hall-McCorquodale investigated the incidence of mother-blaming in major clinical journals and identified 77 different problems (emotional as well as physical) as attributable to mothers. What is particularly interesting is that they reviewed journals for the years 1970, 1976, and 1982 in order to determine whether any reductions resulted from the efforts of the women's movement. They found very few changes longitudinally. In addition, mother-blaming was only slightly affected by the sex of the author, that is, women were only slightly less likely to engage in mother-blaming.

While mothers are usually blamed for the mental illness suffered by their children, they continue to be burdened by caregiving responsibilities. Eckholm (1986) in the *New York Times* states: "Often the mothers carry the heaviest loads. In a familiar syndrome, the mother accepts the child's condition as an illness while the father persists in seeing it as misbehavior requiring discipline." In the same article, quoting a parent, "It's not uncommon for the father to segregate himself from the problem. We see a lot of women attending support group meetings whose husbands refuse to come, or have left them."

How have nurses working in mental health perceived and interacted with the mothers of the chronically mentally ill regarding mother-blaming? As members of a profession made up almost entirely of women, nurses initially appear to be in a position that prompts them to be empathic to the experiences of mothers. Nurses and mothers are in similar caregiving roles, and like mothers, nurses are frequently responsible for the 24-hour care of clients.

Fagin and Diers (1983) describe nursing as a repository for "metaphor." Two of the metaphors they identify are nursing as a metaphor for mothering and for class struggle.

> *Nursing has links with nurturing, caring, comforting, the laying on of hands, and other maternal types of behavior, . . . Not only does nursing represent women's struggles for equality, but its position in the health world is that of classic underdog, struggling to be heard, approved and recognized. . . . They work predominately in settings that are dominated by physicians and in which physicians represent the upper and controlling class.* (p. 116)

Roberts (1983), in her discussion of oppressed group behavior and its implications for nursing, describes behaviors that develop in oppressed groups.

Those oppressed internalize the values of the dominant culture. The oppressed individual wishing to attain power or status becomes more like the oppressor.

The dominant group in a culture identifies and enforces the "correct" values of a society. Mental health nurses work with psychiatrists, mostly men and thus members of the dominant group. Covertly or overtly, their characteristics as nurses and women often become negatively valued.

Dynamics of oppressed group behavior indicate that, rather than entering into an empathic relationship with mothers, nurses are more likely to identify with the oppressor and enter into and maintain a passive or conflictual relationship with mothers.

Therefore, it is imperative that nurses working in the area of mental health examine the attitudes of the "dominant group" toward the mother of the mentally ill son or daughter. A historical perspective must be gained to understand the present context of mothers and nurses as interacting members of the mental health team.

Within the mental health system mothers have been viewed as causative agents. Although one could return to the misogynist climate of witch hunts and the *Malleus Maleficarum* to identify an appropriate paradigm for mother-blaming, there is no need to look further back than this century.

Schizophrenia and bipolar illness were being categorized as disease entities at the turn of the century. A medical model, with emphasis on organic and neurophysiological causality, was prevalent at that time.

But soon thereafter, Freud, a neurologist, initiated the paradigmatic shift from biological to intrapsychic etiologies. As the founder of psychoanalysis, Freud asserted that early infant experiences laid the groundwork for personality development. Thus began the examination of mothering as a causal agent of mental disorders.

Chodorow (1978) explains that mothers are viewed as having responsibility for both physological and psychological care of their offspring. According to the psychoanalytic perspective, a child's successful completion of the developmental process of separating from mother and gaining independence depends on the mother providing nurturance while carefully avoiding overprotection or rejection.

Maternal style as a causal influence in the development of mental disorders is evidenced most strikingly by the coining of the term "schizophrenogenic mother" by Frieda Fromm-Reichmann in 1949. A practicing psychoanalyst, Fromm-Reichmann stated

> *The schizophrenic is painfully distrustful and resentful of other people, due to the severe early warp and rejection he encountered in important people of his infancy and childhood, as a rule, mainly in a schizophrenic mother.* (p. 265)

The evolution of the concept of the "schizophrenogenic mother" in the literature was reviewed by Parker in 1982. He cites numerous clinical studies, as far back as 1934, that identify a dominant, overprotective but basically rejecting mother as the causal influence in the development of schizophrenia. Frank (1965) also reviewed numerous studies that portray the mother of the schizophrenic as being dominant and intrusive. Although most of these studies seem to equate mothering with parenting, many studies also include the role of father as influencing psychopathology. Essentially, the father is described as being passive and ineffectual. Although this doesn't exactly absolve the father, his could be considered a sin of omission. In addition, until quite recently, fathers' responsibility for parenting was viewed as being secondary to the many other social roles he fulfills (Chodorow, 1978).

These studies were first cited in the psychoanalytic literature but by the end of World War II American psychiatry was characterized by a radical environmentalism (Beck, Rawlins, & Williams, 1968). Not only were psychoanalysts interested in looking at early development but social scientists were investigating family and social milieus. Emerging models included systems model, communication model, and family interactionalist model. These models are not easily distinguished from each other. But Torrey (1988) illuminates the actual change which occurred in regard to families being causal agents:

> These family interactional theories were a direct offspring of the psychoanalysts, but in place of what-mother-did-to-baby-at-six-months were introduced concepts about what-mother-said-to-son-at-age-12. (p. 163)

For example, Bateson et al. (1956) developed the "double-bind" theory of schizophrenia. They asserted that the thought disorder seen in the schizophrenic is caused by the child being placed in a "no win" situation in their interactions with parents, especially the mother. Case studies of the "double-bind" theory describing how interactions are played out in the family nearly always use the mother–son dyad. The father is usually portrayed as remaining passive and failing to make any intervention. Once again father is characterized as being less overtly responsible as a causal agent.

It is important to note that most of the family studies of schizophrenia are cross-sectional in design (Reiss, 1980). The family is studied after the onset of the illness and, therefore, the behavior that they exhibit is likely to be seen as the cause of the disorder.

One might question why a mother's domineering style (as well as a father's passivity) was not viewed as being a response to the illness rather than the causal agent. Does it not make sense that a mother would react to the severe behavior changes she finds in her son or daughter? But the notion of family members of the chronically mentally ill being victims of this disease was not reflected in these family studies. Eventually, however, the topic of family burden did emerge.

Beginning in the 1960s, the locus of treatment changed from the institution to the community. Many psychiatric clients were moving home. Newly diagnosed patients were hospitalized for brief periods. The issue of "family burden" became a subject for research. In 1974, Kreisman and Joy reviewed studies that identified sources of family burden as:

> threatening or embarrassing behavior by the patient, the social stigma attached to mental illness, self-blame and guilt experienced by parents, the financial strain of treatment, the marital disruption caused by the illness, and the parent's responsibility to provide extensive supervision for the patient. (p. 36)

Families found the mental health system unresponsive to their needs and the needs of their relative. Parents were experiencing both shame and blame. When they sought treatment the blame was only reinforced. As one father stated (Eckholm, 1986), "We paid people $75 an hour to tell us it was our fault. We believed them and that kept us in the closet."

This lack of response to family needs and reinforcement of guilt within parents led to the emergence around the country of activism on the part of families of the mentally disturbed. The National Alliance for the Mentally Ill is the most notable result of this activism movement. Since 1979, the National Alliance for the Mentally Ill has grown from 80 local family groups to over 600. The goals of this "family movement" are emotional support, public education and advocacy of neglected programs, and research on severe mental diseases, schizophrenia foremost among them.

As a result of this activism, researchers within the psychosocial rehabilitation framework began to assess the needs of families by directly asking family members to report their needs. A number of studies examined family needs, family perceptions of the responsiveness of mental health professionals to meet these needs, and the perceptions of mental health professionals to the needs of families and their goals when treating the chronically mentally ill.

Spaniol, Zipple, and Fitzgerald (1984a) found that families need information about mental illness, as well as assistance in the management of psychiatric symptoms, problematic behavior, and medications. He also identified that families need assistance with coping with stress.

Studies that examined family perceptions as to whether these needs were met by mental health professionals indicated that families are "generally dissatisfied with mental health professionals, families do not generally find them helpful, and, in fact often feel blamed by them for the disability of their mentally ill relative" (Spaniol & Zipple, 1984b).

In 1984, Spaniol performed a national survey that assessed coping strategies of families of the mentally ill. His results indicate that, despite being stressed, burdened, and overwhelmed in the caregiving role, families have a broad range of coping strategies that they report to be effective. "They are needy but not helpless."

Hatfield (1984) asked mental health professionals about their perceptions of goals for treatment and the needs of families. The result indicated a misperception of the needs of families and a resistance to focus on the needs identified by families.

In the early 1980s, partially in response to the activism of family members and the emergence (reemergence?) of biological models of causation, a psychoeducational approach emerged to working with families of the mentally ill. This approach attempts to engage the family in a partnership and gives the family some sense of control. In addition, in this approach there is no blame placed on the family for causing the illness.

It is now quite obvious that the mental health system has been slow to meet the needs of the families of the mentally ill. For most of this century the focus has been on "blaming" rather than providing support and education. Changes in this system have been motivated by a family self-help movement rather than from within the system. Mothers, who have endured the process of being blamed and demoralized, have eventually gained empowerment through mutual support and education.

Therefore, there is a need to move toward a more comprehensive, pragmatic approach to assisting clients and their families. Although this might not meet the professionals' needs for conducting insight-oriented therapy, it decreases the incongruencies that plague the system.

In the assessment of attitudes of mental health professionals within the psychosocial rehabilitation literature, nurses, strangely or not so strangely, were not delineated as a category. In the same sense, it is not clear what family perceptions are regarding the responsiveness of nurses in meeting their needs.

To determine the role of nurses and their attitudes toward parents of the chronically mentally ill, particularly mothers, I examined the nursing literature. First, I reviewed a sampling of psychiatric nursing textbooks, the rationale being that these are the learning tools that introduce nursing students to the field of mental health nursing.

In 1984, Osborne reported on his review of the intellectual traditions in psychiatric mental health nursing through a review of selected textbooks. He states, "Textbooks are more than teaching devices. They are historical and political statements" (p. 31). He adds that as political statements they have faltered.

I reviewed eight psychiatric nursing textbooks published from 1983 to 1988 (Beck, Rawlins, & Williams, 1988; Burgess, 1985; Johnson, 1986; Kreigh & Perko, 1983; Murray & Huelskoetter, 1987; Norris, et al. 1987; Stuart & Sundeen, 1987; Wilson & Kneisl, 1988). I examined each for two primary aspects: presentation of the causative factors of schizophrenia and coverage of family issues in regard to schizophrenia, especially relating to the needs of the chronically mentally ill.

The majority of these texts described a number of theories, including psychosocial and biological. For the most part, psychosocial theories are presented in a neutral manner with no commentary as to how they may or may not impact on the family.

In regard to psychoanalytic theories, I found covert, rather than overt, mother-blaming. Frieda Fromm-Reichmann, originator of the "schiziophrenigenic mother" concept, is identified in more than one text as a contributor to psychoanalytic thinking.

A number of texts discuss the double-bind theory. In almost all cases the mother is presented as the parent giving the double message.

Each of the texts draws the conclusion that causality is multifactored and is most likely a combination of psychosocial and biological factors. Most texts do not mention that the majority of clients will return home.

Wilson and Kneisl (1988), in their recently released third edition, are the first to clearly refute dysfunctional family interaction as a causative factor of schizophrenia. As the edition just mentioned, Beck (1988) also has distinct chapters for discussion of the chronically mentally ill. However, Wilson and Kneisl clearly address the issue of family burden. These authors also state "some mental health professionals have a bias against family involvement" (p. 415).

Essentially, this review of texts indicates, for the most part, an attempt at neutrality in the presentation of theories of causation and a lack of substance in regard to the needs of families.

In addition to exploring psychiatric nursing textbooks, I reviewed psychiatric nursing journals. Journals are the voices which communicate the latest, most salient issues in a field.

I found a paucity of work that address the issues of the role of nurses and their attitudes toward the parents of the chronically mentally ill. Although some articles address issues related to the chronically mentally ill, such as medication compliance and specific treatment strategies, focus on family needs was lacking. Exceptions, of course, do exist.

In a 1983 article in the British *Journal of Advanced Nursing* entitled "Understanding Mental Illness: The Experience of Families of Psychiatric

Patients," Rose and her colleagues through a qualitative study elicited the families perceptions of their experience of the first hospitalization of a relative. Unstructured interviews, conducted in the families' homes focused on events leading to hospitalization including hospital admission, perceptions of the hospital environment, perceptions of the treatment received by the patient, and the effect of hospitalization on their everyday lives. Rose describes one family member's experience.

> When a person has a . . . goes into a hospital ward, has an accident in a car, goes into a hospital and they're going to do certain things, there's a punctured lung and there's this and there's that, they take you aside and they say, "now this is what the situation is and this is what we're going to do . . ."

The family member went on to describe how he wanted and expected this kind of information regarding his relative's situation, but did not receive it.

Such lack of information forthcoming from staff made it difficult for families to understand the meaning of the treatments, and the meaning of mental illness. Rose (1983) adds that nurses need to be aware of the stress experienced by families.

> Families blame themselves. Nurses and others working with families should be sensitive to this process of families examining their own behavior. They should be ready to anticipate and receive questions about causality and they should be aware of any indirect messages they may give to families when interacting with them. (p. 511)

Rose concludes that "an acceptable attitude and a supportive environment are necessary if we expect families to share their feelings and beliefs" (p. 511).

A 1985 article by the same author and her colleagues at the University of British Columbia, entitled "Group Support for the Families of Psychiatric Patients," in the *Journal of Psychosocial Nursing*, describes a study of the use of professionally led support groups. Two of the authors, both nurses, used an exploratory design to determine how a support group for families of psychiatric patients could help them deal with related problems and concerns. Initially, group members focused on the ill relative and the difficulties obtaining help from the health care system. The focus then progressed to expression of guilt, worry, and sadness. The outcome of the group was that the families gained strength and confidence in their management of their relatives' illness, including how to get help from professionals. The authors conclude that this nursing intervention is a "powerful and effective means of meeting the needs of families during the hospitalization phase of the patient's illness" (p. 29).

This review of mental health nursing textbooks and journals indicates that overt mother-blaming in the nursing care of the chronically mentally ill is not documented. In addition, there is generally a lack of documentation of the families of the chronically mentally ill and about nurses' relationships with the mothers of the mentally ill.

The psychosocial rehabilitation literature, as well as Rose's contributions, indicate that, in general, mental health professionals do not meet the needs of the families of concern. In fact, mental health professionals rarely understand the needs of family members, especially mothers.

This lack of focus on the informal caregivers of the chronically mentally ill in both nursing journals and textbooks indicates, at best, a passive attitude toward these caregivers. This apathetic response reflects oppressed group behavior. Nurse researchers and authors have joined the dominant group and negated the needs of mothers of the mentally ill. Nurses who are direct caregivers, while sharing with mothers of the chronically mentally ill a culture of caregiving, have failed to align themselves with these mothers.

Clearly, nurses need to look at what can be done to improve their future relationship with mothers who care for a chronically mentally ill son or daughter. Education and research are two areas that must be considered.

Freire (1970, 1973), however, sees education as one of the mechanisms used by a culture to reinforce the myths of the dominant group. Freire speaks to a "banking concept" of education in which the teacher's role is to make "deposits" into passive students. Are the encyclopedic textbooks found in nursing today, with their lack of critical commentary, reflective of this "banking concept" of education?

Freire sees the potential to move to a more reciprocal form of education, an education of freedom. Hedin (1986), a nursing scholar, describes this education of freedom. She states

> a freeing education allows the participants to move to a level of critical consciousness . . . which is characterized by the attitude of practicing depth in the interpretation of problems. (p. 54)

Nurse educators must encourage students to understand what mothers experience in caring for their children. One way educators can facilitate this process is to invite mothers of the chronically ill into the classroom to tell their stories to students, thereby giving their experiences a voice.

Most importantly, as a means of fostering critical thinking and improving caring interactions in the clinical setting, nursing educators must uncover the dynamics of oppression that can occur within nursing.

In nursing research, there is need to understand the meaning of experiences of mothers of the chronically mentally ill. Qualitative research methods can be useful in meeting this need. A feminist perspective offers methodologies that seek to gain an understanding of the female experience (Duffy, 1985). These methods call for equal status to exist between the researcher and the subjects. This is research for women aimed at the political and social change needed in the mental health system. The prevailing relationship of "power over" others that the system fosters must be changed to "power within" caregivers, especially within nurses and mothers.

Mental health nurses need to construct theories that will dramatically alter the oppressive structures and practices that undermine our caregiving potential.

REFERENCES

Anderson, C. M., Hogarty, G. E., & Reiss, D. J. (1980). Family treatment of adult schizophrenic patients: A psycho-educational approach. *Schizophrenia Bulletin 6*, 490–505.

Arieti, S. (1984). *Interpretation of schizophrenia* (2nd edition). New York: Basic Books.

Bateson, G., Jackson, D. D., Haley, J., & Weakland, J. (1956). Toward a theory of schizophrenia. *Behavioral Science 1*, 251–263.

Beck, C. K., Rawlins, R. P., & Williams, S. R. (1988). *Mental health-psychiatric nursing: A holistic life-cycle approach*. St. Louis: C. V. Mosby.

Burgess, A. W. (1985). *Psychiatric nursing in the hospital and community* (4th edition). Englewood Cliffs, NJ: Prentice-Hall.

Caplan, P., & Hall-McCorquodale, I. (1985). Mother-blaming in major clinical journals. *American Journal of Orthopsychiatry 55*(3) 345–353.

Carper, B. A. (1978). Fundamental patterns of knowing in nursing. *Advances in Nursing Science 1*(1), 13–23.

Duffy, M. (1985). A critique of research: A feminist perspective. *Health Care for Women International 6*, 341–352.

Eckholm, E. (1986). Schizophrenia's victims include strained families. *New York Times*. March 17, 1986.

Fagin, C., & Diers, D. (1983). Nursing as metaphor. *New England Journal of Medicine 309*, 116–117.

Freire, P. (1970). *Pedagogy of the oppressed* (M. B. Ramos, Trans.). New York: Continuum Press.

Freire, P. (1973). *Education for critical consciousness.* (Center for the Study of Development and Social Change, Trans.). New York: Continuum Press.

Fromm-Reichmann, F. (1948). Notes on the development and treatment of schizophrenics by psychoanalytic psychotherapy. *Psychiatry 2,* 263–273.

Goldman, H. H. (1982). Mental illness and family burden; a public health perspective. *Hospital and Community Psychiatry 33,* 557–559.

Hatfield, A. (1984). *Coping with mental illness in the family: The family guide.* Arlington, VA: National Alliance of the Mentally Ill.

Hedin, B. (1986). A case study of oppressed group behavior in nurses. *Image 18*(2), 53–57.

Johnson, B. S. (1986). *Psychiatric-mental health nursing: Adaptation and growth.* Philadelphia: J. B. Lippincott.

Kanter, J., Lamb, H. R., & Loeper, C. (1987). Expressed emotion in families: A critical review. *Hospital and Community Psychiatry, 38*(4), 374–380.

Kreigh, H. Z., & Perko, J. E. (1983). *Psychiatric and mental health nursing: A commitment to care and concern.* (2nd edition). Reston, VA: Reston Publishing Company.

Kreisman, D. E., & Joy, V. D. (1974). Family response to the mental illness of a relative: A review of the literature. *Schizophrenia Bulletin, 10,* 34–57.

Murray, R. B., & Huelskoetter, M. M. (1987). *Psychiatric/mental health nursing: Giving emotional care.* (2nd edition). Norwalk, CT: Appleton and Lange.

Norris, J., Kunes-Connell, M., Stockard, S., Ehrhart, P. M., & Newton, G. R. (1987). *Mental health-psychiatric nursing: A continuum of care.* New York: John Wiley and Sons.

Osborne, O. H. (1984). Intellectual traditions in psychiatric mental health nursing: a review of selected textbooks. *Journal of Psychosocial Nursing 22*(11), 27–32.

Parker, G. (1982). Re-searching the schizophrenogenic mother. *The Journal of Nervous and Mental Disease, 170*(8), 452–462.

Reiss, D. (1980). Pathways to assessing the family: Some choice points and sample route. In C. K. & Lewis, J. M. (Eds.), *The family: evaluation and treatment.* New York: Brunner Mazel.

Roberts, S. J. (1983). Oppressed group behavior: Implications for nursing. *Advances in Nursing Science, 5*(4), 21–30.

Rose, L. (1983). Understanding mental illness: The experience of families of psychiatric patients. *Journal of Advanced Nursing, 8,* 507–511.

Rose, L., Finestone, K., & Bass, J. (1985). Group support for the families of psychiatric patients. *Journal of Psychosocial Nursing, 23*(12), 24–29.

Sederer, L. (1987). *Inpatient psychiatry: Diagnosis and treatment.* (2nd edition) Baltimore: Williams and Wilkins.

Spaniol, L., Zipple, A. M., & Fitzgerald, S. (1984a). How professionals can share power with families: A practical approach to working with families of the mentally ill. *Psychosocial Rehabilitation Journal, 8*(2), 77–84.

Spaniol, L., & Zipple, A. (1984b). *Current research on families that include a person with a severe mental illness: A review of the findings.* Available from The Center for Rehabilitation Research and Training in Mental Health, Boston University.

Stuart, G. W., & Sundeen, S. J. (1987). *Principles and practice of psychiatric nursing.* (3rd edition). St. Louis: C. V. Mosby.

Terkelson, K. G. (1983). Schizophrenia and the family. *Family Process, 22,* 191–200.

Tietze, T. (1949). A study of mothers of schizophrenic patients. *Psychiatry, 12,* 55–65.

Torrey, E. F. (1988). *Surviving schizophrenia: A family manual* (revised edition). New York: Harper & Row.

Wilson, H., & Kneisl, C. (1988). *Psychiatric nursing* (3rd edition). Reading, MA: Addison-Wesley Publishing Company.

13

Codependency: Caring or Suicide for Nurses and Nursing?

Nina A. Klebanoff

INTRODUCTION

Because of their role as caregivers and the predominance of women in the profession of nursing, nurses can be expected to exhibit a high incidence and extreme severity of codependency and internalized oppression. In addition, the essential character and the practice of nursing—as well as its position in the power structure of the techno-medico-industrial complex—reveals a perfect profile of codependency/internalized oppression. This constitutes a serious occupational hazard for nursing as a profession and for nurses as individuals. By recognizing these influences, nurses can address the problems from a systematic perspective and begin to find ways to counteract their pervasive and debilitating effects.

CONCEPTS AND CONTEXT

To suggest the special significance of codependency to female nurses through a feminist analysis of the relationship among codependency, internalized oppression, feminism, and caring involves an examination of the similarities among the concepts. These concepts indicate that nurses are at high risk of integrating/adopting unhealthy self-regard and nurse–client and professional relationship patterns since all three of these influences operate simultaneously and synergistically.

Because nurses and nursing dwell in a patriarchal milieu, nurses must be skillful at holding and balancing several belief systems in awareness at once. For example, we often choose an effective combination of nursing and medical approaches to provide client care in any of the many settings in which we practice.

From a feminist perspective, sexism and codependency are inextricably linked. Sexism, a symptom and form of patriarchy, is a system largely controlled by white males. Patriarchy, of course, largely defines the dominant culture we live in and the structure of obedience we are conditioned to behave in accord with. Unfortunately, patriarchal values are based on dominance and subordination, and other values otherwise indicative of male white supremacy with an emphasis on control and separation.

The profession of nursing itself reveals a microcosm of patriarchal society reflected in and serving as a magnifying mirror. Under the looking glass we can "see" primarily male or male-identified physicians and administrators as lord-master-father, overwhelmingly female nurses as slave-servant-mother with patients/clients/consumers as objects or subhuman children. We live in a culture where it is "normal" to have come from a dysfunctional family; it is estimated that 80 percent of nurses are codependent (Black, 1981; Woitiz, 1985). This has profound repercussions for the self-image of nurses and the public image of nursing.

The phenomenal success of Robin Norwood's (1985) book, *Women Who Love Too Much,* (is it possible to love too much?) and the proliferation of support groups based on that book testify to the resonance women experience regarding codependency. This raises the question: Is codependency a peculiarly female affliction? Certainly the syndrome is as old as the patriarchy (at least five thousand years), but until five to seven years ago it had no definition. The recent naming of codependency has helped thousands, if not millions, of us to understand underlying patterns in our relationships.

As a concept, codependency originated in psychotherapies, notably family systems, and modalities treating addiction and substance abuse. Nonaddicted partners were described as exhibiting "codependent" behavior as their lives revolved around their partner's illness. Therapists found that codependency persisted after the primary addiction was treated and realized that the syndrome required separate treatment. At that time, the term *codependency* did not carry any gender associations. But as the term has been extended to include a wide range of unhealthy, obsessive patterns of intimacy, it has acquired a gender link.

There are as many definitions of codependency as there are authors who discuss the phenomenon. For example, definitions range from Larson (1985) who states that codependency is caused by those self-defeating, learned behaviors that diminish our capacity to initiate or participate in loving relationships to Cermak (1986) establishing diagnostic criteria for "codependent personality disorder." The symptoms and behavior indicative of codependency also run the gamut from being too loyal and assuming too much responsibility for others to suicide and psychosis. Many caring, compassionate traits and behaviors resemble definitions of codependency. Defined here, codependency is a set of survival skills for living in the patriarchy, that is, dealing with internalized oppression. At one and the same time it provides defense against the patriarchy while being used by the patriarchy to label and define (as well as encourage self-definition of) the handmaidens and "victims" of the dominant system. As a label and a method of social control, codependency is the witch-burning of our present times.

Internalized oppression is a mechanism by which one takes the values of and from the dominant culture, thereby ensuring the continuance of that culture or system. A crucial factor in the successful maintenance of patriarchal society, which is based on dominance and subordination, is internalized oppression. Through this intimate enforcement system, the target or victim of oppression incorporates and introjects the dominant values, such as inferiority of women to men, blacks to whites, or nurses to physicians. In our case, the nurse accepts her oppression as inevitable and constantly references the oppressor's needs before her own in order to survive and protect the client. This acceptance and practice of other-referencing results in a constricted emotional range and a zealous effort to care for others. The Internal Decision Cycle (Hagan, 1987), which can circularly reinforce the patriarchy, illustrates the progression of internalized oppression.

The Internal Decision Cycle

There are seven steps to the Internal Decision Cycle:

1. The Frame of Reference or Belief System.

2. The Program.

3. The Conditioning.

4. The Habit or Pattern.

5. The Daily Day.

6. The Choice/Action.

7. The Synap.

To begin with, it is the last step which becomes the first step in the ever-repeating cycle. The Synap is the nanopause between receiving sensory and intuitive input and translating it into step one, the Frame of Reference or Belief System. It is in this last aspect of the cycle that we can alter the direction of our lives.

In the context of nursing, the Frame of Reference is established by the Belief System of the dominant culture. In this case, the Belief System includes the assumption that the nurse/doctor/patient pattern is modeled after the patriarchal marriage and the nuclear family. In short, nurses are the "wife" and "mother" in the triad with physicians as the "husband" and "father" and role of the "children" falls to the clients and all other staff and employees (Ashley, 1976). Father is the head of the family in which the children have token rights and the mothers are the "token torturers" (Daly, 1978, pp. 276-277). A myth of the holy marriage (Ashley, 1976) is acted out in this relationship between the male medical profession and the female nursing profession. Nursing exemplifies the workplace extension of the role of women in the dominant society, that is, as wife (to care for physicians) and as mother (to care for patients and staff members) (Ehrenreich & English, 1973).

The second step in the cycle, the Program, is a conceptual framework or blueprint of the set of values undergirding the Frame of Reference. The foundation of the patriarchy is based on values such as, but not limited to, dominance, control, coercion, dehumanization, deception, and exploitation. If nurses follow the Program, then success in the patriarchy is enhanced. For example, we will serve physicians, hate ourselves, and sacrifice our lives for others to create an acceptable "family." We do this as necessary to the next step, the Conditioning.

The Conditioning is the behavioral reinforcement upholding the Program. We are rewarded for our obedience to the patriarchy and punished for disobedience. Assertive nurses are ridiculed. This and other "gestures of dominance" (Daly, 1978) support the system we live in. That nurses assault each other (horizontal violence) covertly and overtly is to be expected as conditioned in a patriarchal Frame of Reference and Program.

The Habit or Pattern is the specific "evidence of our individual behavior following the hidden agenda over time" (Hagan, 1987). The Habit or Pattern, determined by the choices we make, is a sequence of behaviors that chip away at our self-esteem. Whenever we choose to act in such a way as to "protect against a lawsuit" or "cover for the doctor" at the direct or indirect expense of our own integrity or the welfare of a client or family or community, we reinforce the Habit or Pattern. We do this in the course of living our Daily Day.

The Daily Day is the setting or context in which we carry out, systematically and chronically, the embedded values of our culture. For example, the setting of the Daily Day for a majority of nurses is the hierarchical, business-medico-centered hospital. In the course of a Daily Day we make innumerable decisions to decide; Choice/Action ensues during the Daily Day.

The moment of intention or decision instantly precedes the Choice/Action. That is, the internal value and belief system becomes an external act. The sequence of Choice/Action later creates our Habits or Patterns. We have all heard of and lived stories as nurses who have "automatically" risen and given their seats to the doctor on his or her arrival. This step in the Internal Decision Cycle feeds into the Synap.

The Linkages

When we examine the process of decision making, we can see how internalized oppression manifests itself. We direct our energy to support our belief and value systems. If we hold that nurses are inferior, then we will act in a manner which supports that notion. Internalized oppression affects and molds our core beliefs. If, conversely, we believe that nurses are worthy of respect, we will act accordingly.

In other words, changing our consciousness to support patriarchal values is internalized oppression. If we are contrary to our own will, or believe that our own will is better served by obeying the will of the patriarchy, then we do not have to be controlled by physical bonds or in prisons. Besides, such forms of social control are labor intensive, costly, and create public relations problems for the patriarchy (as is the case in South Africa). Internalized oppression is a more attractive, cost-effective, and convenient form of social control; and it is all but invisible (Hagan, 1987). Implicitly we are controlled by the reality or the threat of rape, incest, and child abuse and punishment, which are construed to be our own fault anyway.

A feminist scrutiny of codependency reveals a striking similarity between the characteristics of codependency and internalized oppression, such as external referencing, poor self-esteem, martyrhood (self-righteousness which leads to resentment), controlling behavior (helping and fixing those who can do so for themselves), and rapid as well as pervasive demoralization. Both the codependent individual and the victim of internalized oppression derive self-worth primarily through being needed by others.

Patriarchal values are constantly reinforced by institutions, laws, customs, the media, and personal and professional interactions. We become our own oppressors by internalizing tho e values. Our conditioned internal voices then reinforce the patriarchal values based on dominance and subordination. Feminism is a Frame of Reference that presents an alternative to the dominant patriarchal worldview.

FEMINISM

Feminism is a world view which advocates all life forms without exploiting any while embracing diversity and interconnection. Beliefs and habits that respect and encourage self-loving, respect for nature, creativity, integrity, and that foster interconnection with others are feminist in nature. Daly (1984) and Daly and Caputi (1987) provides us with the following tenets of radical feminism:

1. A presence of intuitive feeling of otherness. A self-reflection that is alien to the patriarchal worldview and connected with nature.
2. The real knowledge of the oppressive sanctions that bear on women (and children) from the patriarchy.
3. A deep sense of moral outrage on behalf of women as women. Coupled with that sense is a past, present, and future woman-identified perspective.
4. A constant companion in life where relationship to self will flourish.

A brief examination of the economic, political, social, and professional aspects of contradicting the grain of codependency will follow. From this, a discussion of the potential impact of shifting to a feminist from a patriarchal paradigm on the local, state, national and international arenas will evolve.

Implications and Impact

We live in an addictive society (Schaef, 1987). If, as has been estimated, more than 90 percent of all American families are dysfunctional, that must be the norm, what is typical in patriarchal society. For example, the economic arrangement of the current dominant culture is shown by the fact that nurses (women) make less than 70 cents for every one dollar that a man makes. We are all too familiar with the relative lack of political power that nurses have. As nurses, we are aware of the social costs, such as violence, illness, disease, divorce, hunger, and homelessness, to name a few. The professional implications are vast. These range from nonexistent to inhibited collaboration and parity with other professionals to not being aware of the activities of nurses in other countries on other continents.

Because patriarchal values exist on a global scale, we are an estranged, lonely, and competitive people. If feminism were to "replace" the patriarchal world we live in, effects would ripple throughout the local, state, and international communities. The diminishment and evaporation of the acts and effects of sexism, rape, incest, child and elder abuse, and others which cannot be anticipated beforehand are hypothesized in a feminist framework.

The patriarchal framework and value system assigns inferiority to the oppressed (and codependent) and ensures that the patriarchy continues. Oppression theory and feminist theory have provided the frameworks for analysis of codependency as it impacts on nurses and nursing. Self-observation and "reprogramming" assist the paradigm shift toward a more life-affirming world. Nurses have been "trained" to sacrifice themselves. That phenomenon is not an individual shortcoming or disease. Nurses and nursing are not sick, bad, or to blame. Rather, society is responsible for the socialization (read: conditioning) provided to its members. Individual nurses (and professional nursing), however, must now take responsibility for the resultant thoughts, behaviors, and feelings. Hagan (1987) states, "It is in this intimate setting of personal decision making that the most important step of societal change is made."

PERSONAL/PROFESSIONAL INVOLVEMENT: WHAT TO DO

Awareness that we have a choice at the point prior to the Frame of Reference (at the Synap) in the Internal Decision Cycle is liberating. This can be anticipated or done spontaneously. However, it is sometimes useful during transition phases or for matters of personal safety to be consciously codependent on a selective basis. However, once we allow ourselves to consider that the patriarchy is not immutable or eternal, we open ourselves to other possibilities of individual development; there is much more than what we were taught and what we were offered as far as worldviews and ways of relating to ourselves and each other. Because the patriarchy presents in and is the foreground (Connors, 1976) of prevailing cultural norms, it invests much time, effort, and money to create and maintain the illusion of its hegemony. Yet when we stop and listen to our own authority, our own natural, elemental wisdom enables us to see through to the background.

As such, we can change our internal voices since they belong to us. According to Hagan (1987), "Increasing our awareness, of our conditioning and of the possibilities beyond it, can change the way we live our daily lives." This can be accomplished by observing and comparing it (and conditioning) with our actual experience, thereby reclaiming our personal needs, desires, and vision of how the world could be. Thus, we enter into an intentional, willful, growing process that dismantles the hold of internalized oppression and moves beyond patriarchy. By naming what we want and envisioning the ideal—a spiritual expression—we can set goals and chart directions of our own volition.

We can embark on a journey to teach ourselves and others how to be free and include more options. We can start to re-teach and re-program what we have been taught in a culture which generally proscribes against the development of independent women (theoretically) free of patriarchal structures. Marilyn Frye (1983) provides an example of the draft animal to teach us about learning how to set ourselves free. Draft animals have been transgenerationally conditioned to pull plows to the extent that their anatomy is transmogrified so that they can do work more efficiently. If one day you decide to set a draft horse free, and take the harness off of it, what happens? By itself the act means little. The horse knows one thing: to stand there as before. Learning how to be free does not come easily. Living freely is a conscious, deliberate, and intentional activity, which takes patience, practice, and perseverance.

If we as nurses (women) stop, widen our frame of reference and value system to align ourselves with our own caring belief system, the entire decision-making process is altered. Nurses can define and claim nursing as an autonomous, healing profession. Nursing is a network of supportive people among whom is a shared vision and commitment to care for others in such a way that affirms, not exploits, people. To live in accordance with this version of connected reality brings about changes in one's daily day and the system.

We each have a responsibility to alter the direction of our lives. We can surpass the restrictive and proscriptive structures of patriarchy. To return to a prior level of functioning, which amounts to further self-blame and victimization, is out of the question. We can discover, create, test, try, evaluate, and employ the nursing process toward "new" and "old" ways of being and relating. Such activity will transform our estrangement, isolation, and disconnection from the self, others, and nature. Finally, such relating might prevent the very harm and destruction of ourselves, others, and our environment so prevalent today.

When we make a change at the level of the Synap, the effect ripples throughout the entire sequence so as to break the set of our core beliefs that perpetuates our internalized oppression (Hagan, 1987). The following is an offering of prescriptions, suggestions, and strategies for defining and transforming ourselves and nursing on our own terms. It is in no particular order, adapted from a myriad of sources, and is by no means exhaustive.

- Read your own mind and listen to your own heart.
- Do not settle for anything less than absolutely everything. (Too much is not enough!)
- Engage in systematic and rigorous efforts to appreciate yourself, other nurses, and our accomplishments unhesitatingly.
- Commit to treat every other female person with complete respect.
- Offer each other high expectations and bestow confidence.

- Read nursing history and women's history and literature to focus attention on the endeavors and achievements of nursing and women, and to teach others about our issues and accomplishments.
- Spend time with each other.
- Have fun!!
- Expect the men in our lives to be informed and active allies.
- Listen to each other—our personal and professional anxieties, hurts, and joys—to facilitate healing and growing.
- Stand up for yourself and anyone else who is put down whenever someone (male or female) is demeaning a female.
- Attend workshops on women's issues and attend professional meetings and support groups.
- Practice speaking and writing about our caring and thinking in ways that are meaningful.
- Read.
- Decide that the way you want to be and are is totally acceptable and female.
- Take action in the world on issues of importance to you.
- Take action in the world on issues involving oppression.
- Learn about how other girls and women, boys and men, and groups are different from us and how they have been oppressed so as to become dependable allies.
- Consider going to therapy or learning movement techniques.
- Share your story with others and allow yourself to experience fully your feelings about it.
- Do self-esteem work like keeping a journal, listening to affirmation tapes, or participating in creative visualization or meditation practices.
- Pay attention to what you pay attention to.
- Nurture yours in an environment which fosters your growth.
- Question authority.
- Assume nothing.
- Think about how to be, not what to do.
- Take risks.
- Look at the CO-DEPENDENT SCREENING ASSESSMENT TEST (Zerwekh, 1987).

CONCLUSION

That many of you are not yet familiar with the term *codependency* either personally or professionally bodes well for the profession of nursing. To date, the term is not pervasively present in the nursing literature. In other circles, codependency is so overused that it has become meaningless at best and destructive at worst, especially for women. From a feminist perspective, the patterns of codependency and the patterns of internalized oppression of women as nurses are profoundly similar. A feminist exploration of these patterns when linked with caring, nurses, and nursing dramatically enhances the healing process.

REFERENCES

Ashley, J. (1976). Nursing power: Viable, vital, visible. *Texas Nurse*, 50–61.

Black, C. (1981). *It will never happen to me.* Denver: MAC Printing and Publications Division.

Cermak, T. (1986). *Diagnosing and treating co-dependence.* Minneapolis: Johnson Institute Books.

Connors, D. D. (1976, October). Conversation. In M. Daly & J. Caputi (1987), *Webster's first new intergalactic wickedary of the English language.* Boston: Beacon Press.

Daly, M. (1978). *Gyn/ecology: The metaethics of radical feminism.* Boston: Beacon Press.

Daly, M. (1984). *Pure lust: Elemental feminist philosophy.* Boston: Beacon Press.

Daly, M., & Caputi, J. (1987). *Webster's first new intergalactic wickedary of the English language.* Boston: Beacon Press.

Ehrenreich, B., & English, D. (1973). *Witches, midwives and nurses: A history of women healers.* New York: The Feminist Press.

Frye, M. (1983). *The politics of reality: Essays in feminist theory.* Freedom, CA: The Crossing Press.

Hagan, K. (1987). Personal correspondence and interactions seminars and workshop materials. Dallas, Texas.

Larson, E. (1985). *Stage II recovery.* San Francisco: Harper & Row.

Norwood, R. (1985). *Women who love too much.* Los Angeles: Jeremy P. Tarcher, Inc.

Schaef, A. W. (1987). *When society becomes an addict.* San Francisco: Harper & Row.

Woititz, J. G. (1985). *Struggle for intimacy.* Pompano Beach, FL: Health Communications, Inc.

Zerwekh, J. (1987). *Co-Dependent Screening Test Assessment Test (COSAT).* Dallas, Texas.

14

Friendship as a Paradigm for Nursing Science: Using Scientific Subjectivity and Ethical Interaction to Promote Understanding and Social Change

Susan M. Poslusny

Collective insight gathered from the experiences of practicing nurses is important for the profession. In addition, the process that is used to develop that insight, that is, the way that nurses come to know about what they know, is equally important. LeShan and Margenau (1982) propose that domains of knowledge emerge in response to a specific set of problems and that although multiple domains exist, a particular domain is chosen to organize one's thoughts according to what one wants to do. They use the example of appreciating Monet's *Waterlilies*. In one domain the painting is appreciated for its technique, in another for its presumed magnificence. If asked to describe what they saw, an artist and an art collector viewing the same work of art would respond very differently. Similarly, nurses structure and organize their thoughts in a fashion that is appropriate for the problems that they encounter and for the solutions they hope to derive. Paradigms are needed that are relevant to solving nursing problems, and that adequately reflect the process that nurses use in practice to learn, to care, and to discover new information.

In this light, traditional scientific paradigms have been problematic in nursing practice and research. Such paradigms, skewed exclusively toward the perspective of logical positivism, are frequently insufficient to interpret the complex *human* problems encountered by nurses (Watson, 1981). Issues in ethics, interpersonal relations, and quality of care are not reducible to a finite set of variables that can be measured easily, accurately, or completely. There is rarely one "right way" of interpreting nursing problems. Logical positivism helped establish a scientific tradition in nursing, but in the process nursing became estranged from its humanistic tradition.

Scholars in nursing have called for a better "fit" between the philosophy, science, and practice of nursing (Silva, 1977; Munhall, 1982). Recent interest in intuition (Agan, 1987), feminist analysis (MacPherson, 1983; Thompson, 1987), and historicism (Silva & Rothbart, 1983) reflects the attempt of nurses to embrace a nonempiricist tradition in nursing science that focuses on subjectivity, social context, and social change.

One of the basic dilemmas in nursing is how to narrow the gap between technology and ontology; how to approach human existence from a holistic perspective; how to incorporate the scientific tradition in an ontology of human caring; how to heal the social wounds of humanity caused by domination and violence. Precocious pregnancy, malnutrition, and depression are problems that have not been amenable to change using traditional empiricist or technological frameworks that artificially magnify singular dimensions of human experience.

Thus, the questions that prompted this paper were: How do nurses go about discovering new information? Is the process different when the focus of discovery is abstract conceptualization versus interpersonal relations? Can subjective perspective, such as intuition and personal experience, be acknowledged as it contributes to knowledge seeking and concept development? How can values influence science in a way that goes beyond "does no harm." In considering these questions, I was reminded of the very traditional ethic of professionalism in nursing.

In the past, professionalism in nursing inferred distance and objectivity in interpersonal relations with others (Robb, 1920; Aiken, 1935; Poslusny, 1989). An air of friendliness was permitted, but caution was advised to preserve the distance required in a "professional relationship." In a sense, "empiricism" had taken hold of professional nursing relationships. Empiricism in nursing created a strict code of etiquette that governed the nurse behavior. Empiricism also taught that only science revealed the "right way" to be a nurse. I propose that nurses and nursing have evolved to a greater tolerance for diversity in science and practice, and for a new paradigm that is based on interaction, caring, and subjectivity rather than observation, distance, and objectivity.

This paper invokes a metaphor of friendship to describe a new way of thinking about nursing phenomena and nursing practice that incorporates subjective knowledge gained through interaction into a scientific perspective that seeks understanding and social change. Two assumptions distinguish the paradigm: (1) subjectivity is an appropriate, scientific perspective, and (2) science in nursing is best served by a subjectivist perspective that contributes to complete understanding, collective strength, and social change.

The paradigm attempts to integrate the humanistic and scientific traditions of the profession within a context of ethical interaction and scientific subjectivity. Within this perspective nursing is defined as an interactive profession that functions within a social context to promote understanding and effect social change. The nurse uses a subjective awareness of the patient's experience to effect healing, learning, growth, and empowerment. The nurse also abides by an ethic of friendship that is based on the values of care, accountability, and truth. The paradigm blends the themes of feminism and caring into a philosophy that expresses itself through the metaphor of friendship.

The proposed model (see Figure 1) is conceptualized as a web that is joined with strands of empathy learned from the lived experience of individuals. It is a web based on meaningful and ethical interaction reflecting values of care, accountability, and truth. Each nexus represents an interaction. Experience then is the reflection of multiple interactions such that a socially constructed web of relationships is created. Persons share the experience, the meaning associated with each interaction, and the strength derived from the association. Within this conceptualization, nursing science emphasizes increased

Figure 1
Friendship Model for Nursing Science

	ANTECEDENTS	PROCESS	OUTCOMES
S	CARING		
U		LIVED	UNDERSTANDING
B		EXPERIENCE	SOCIAL CHANGE
J		• meeting	• healing
E		• engaging	• learning
C	ACCOUNTABILITY	• connecting	• growth
T			• empowerment
I			
V	TRUTH		
I			
T			
Y	←——————— ETHICAL INTERACTION ————————→		

subjectivity, a focus on lived experience, and ethical interaction. The outcome is mutual understanding and the potential to effect social change from a position of collective strength.

BACKGROUND

Feminism

Feminism brings several major perspectives to the development of this paradigm: emphasis on subjectivity, lived experience, and contextual analysis (McBride & McBride, 1982; Fine, 1985). Postmodern feminism challenges the notions of universality, scientific objectivity, and rationality (Keller, 1985; Harding, 1986). Diversity and subjectivity are recognized as contributing to our better understanding of experience and to the impact this understanding may have on political discourse and social change. Emphasis on lived experience of the individual and contextual analysis seeks to accommodate a full range of experience and to avoid premature narrowing of perception to familiar phenomena and standard interpretations. Exclusion of subjective perspective is thought to artificially limit the accurate and complete appreciation of human experience.

Caring

Health and disease have been described as fundamental expressions of personal and cultural meaning. The inquiry into health and disease has two distinct traditions (Grossinger, 1985). The first is the art of healing which is practiced through sympathy and intuition and "usually involves its own difficult training and techniques and parallels the other tradition in requirements of skill and education" (p. 8). The "other" tradition is "technological-scientific medicine" and includes surgery and pharmacology. The tradition of healing integrates the artificially separated concepts of care and cure. However, an interesting feature of caring as presented in nursing literature is its separation from the cure dimension. Despite discussion of the need for holistic paradigms, the separation of care and cure has persisted.

In actuality, caring includes the healing arts as well as intimacy in the professional relationship. A caring professional relationship also includes an ethic of friendship and a standard of responsible behavior. Caring has been conceptualized as a relational expression of human concern (Carper, 1979; Benner & Wrubel, 1989), and a collection of human activities that assist others (Leininger, 1978). Caring has also been described as a moral attitude (Griffin, 1980), and a pattern of moral reasoning exhibited by women (Gilligan, 1982). Thus, caring is an essential dimension of nursing, involving intimate interaction between the nurse and the patient, and the expression of a moral commitment to engender care (Levine, 1977).

ETHICAL INTERACTION

The professional relationship in nursing is based on an ethic of friendship linked with the values of care (Benner & Wrubel, 1989; Levine, 1977), accountability (Fry, 1981), and truth (Bronowski, 1959). Just as friends care for and about each other, act responsibly toward each other, and trust each other to be honest and sincere, nurses care for and about others. However, nurses are accountable not only to the patient and themselves, but to society and the profession. In the professional relationship, trust is joined by the expectation of truthfulness; truthfulness not in the sense of finding the right truth, but in the sense of accurate and complete disclosure. Thus, the ethic of friendship conveys a standard of moral behavior for the nurse. Within an ethic of friendship that includes authenticity, accountability, and care, potential exists for a scientific and humanistic practice of nursing.

Ethical interaction requires a commitment to achieve full understanding and to render direct benefit to individuals and society. Safe and ethical nursing care is administered only in the presence of full and complete appreciation of the client. Social context is critical to understanding the nature of individual experience. The specific nursing activities and outcomes may be slightly different depending on the situation. For example, within the nursing process, nurse and patient may engage in therapeutic interaction toward an outcome of healing. Other outcomes might include learning, growth, or empowerment. The weaving of an ethical, caring relationship as it is experienced by nurses and clients is aptly characterized by the metaphor of friendship.

SCIENTIFIC SUBJECTIVITY

Friendship is an experience shared by individuals that creates a climate of discovery, encourages learning about oneself and others, and creates shared meaning about the world and reality. Friendship involves discovery, learning, and sharing; or meeting, engaging, and connecting.

A meeting is defined as the act of coming together, and to meet is to encounter in experience. Prior associations may be renegotiated in the context of this new experience. Or the absence of prior association may create opportunity for discovery. However, multiple chance meetings can occur without the formation of any association. Therefore, while a climate of discovery occurs when individuals meet in common circumstances, this does not assure discovery of association. To invoke another metaphor, climatic conditions may be present for rain, but that does not assure that it will rain.

Engagement is the act or state of being engaged. To engage is to attract or please, to enter into conflict or become involved. Engagement takes the encounter to the level of association. Insight or discovery has captured one's attention precipitating attraction and possibly conflict. In the process, learning occurs about the individuals involved. Shared experience creates shared meaning.

Connection is defined as a circle of friends or associates; an association with something observed, imagined, or discussed. To connect is to join, unite, or link. The process of connecting creates relationships and networks based on shared meaning and experience.

In practice, the nurse negotiates a relationship with a client by first making acquaintance and then "getting to know" that person. Some of the initial interactions with the client can be very intense due to the critical nature of the illness experience and the unique meaning that each person brings to the encounter. The interactions are complex, involving interrelated sets of experience, offering multiple interwoven layers of interpretation. Each encounter takes the relationship to a new level of association and brings the opportunity for more complete understanding. Empathy is developed.

Using a perspective called *scientific subjectivity*, the nurse develops empathy through the process of interaction. The nurse primarily employs intuition and identification to initially experience the other's world. Multiple interactions help to triangulate and verify the accuracy and truthfulness of initial perceptions. Complete and honest exchange of actual lived experience assure that mutual understanding and meaningfulness are achieved. Thus, theoretical constructions of knowledge and meaning are subjectively developed based on growing understanding and lived experience.

LIVED EXPERIENCE

Lived experience is a perspective in women's health research that employs subjectivity and contextual analysis to effect social change (Fine, 1985; McBride & McBride, 1982). Biases are made explicit and research "subjects" are considered participants in the entire research process. All participants, including the researcher, interact within an ethic of friendship. Lived experience research is consistent with a paradigm of friendship.

The researcher of lived experience would first become acquainted with literature and individuals that would assist the researcher to develop empathy about the lived experience of women. The literature review would appropriately include historical accounts, case studies, anecdotes, epidemiology, and qualitative research, but would not attempt to select theoretical frameworks for an a priori structure to the research process. The researcher would "meet" and "get to know" the women by negotiating their community and environment. Unstructured discussion and semistructured activity focusing on the particular concerns of the women could take place wherever women reside or gather. These shared experiences would be the context for developing shared meaning about living in their particular environment, and would form the base for future, more structured interactions.

Researcher and subject would remain partners in the research endeavor, each contributing insight and direction for the ultimate development and selection of interview schedules or measurement techniques. This step is not the same as a pilot study in which a small sample of subjects are "tested" in order to discover any difficulties in predetermined methodology. "Getting to know" participants is considered a critical step in identifying relevant variables for study, in creating focus for the study, and in implementing methods that are ethical yet have power and precision. A research relationship must be established before the research partners "engage" in intimate exchange of information that will be shared with the scientific community. Ethically, and scientifically according to a paradigm of friendship, only then could the researcher initiate more structured interviews and measurement of quantitative variables.

Connection, the final step, would involve sharing of research results with the participants and the scientific community; the creation of a contextual ring of insight and understanding through discourse. Interaction is an essential feature of each step in the research process. It is the method and the outcome.

CONCLUSION

This paper has advanced a schema for systematizing a mode of inquiry philosophically more congruent with the humanistic traditions of nursing and scientifically more appropriate for the problems faced by nurses. The preceding example focused on a research experience, but the mode of inquiry is equally applicable to practice-based situations. In constructing the conceptual model, the aim was to capture the process of inquiry as it is experienced by practicing nurses whether as scholars, researchers, or clinicians. I obviously assume that subjectivity is an appropriate, scientific perspective. I also assume that science in nursing is best served by a subjectivist perspective that contributes to collective strength and social change.

Nursing is struggling to find the paradigms that are appropriate for a humanistic profession that maintains a strong alliance with scientific tradition. The profession developed parallel to medicine, and adopted the paradigms of science in an effort to establish a reputable foundation for nursing practice and to elevate the status of the profession to that of the behavioral and natural sciences. The belief that "technique" can take the place of the healing arts has been a powerful influence in the discipline. Nonetheless, an empiricist, techno-medical approach to nursing practice is logically incongruent, taken with a holistic philosophy and the practical questions of contemporary nursing practice. I propose that a paradigm of friendship is logically congruent with the philosophic traditions, ethics, and science of nursing.

REFERENCES

Agan, R. D. (1987). Intuitive knowing as a dimension of nursing. *Advances in Nursing Science, 10*, 63–70.

Aiken, C. A. (1935). *Studies in ethics for nurses.* Philadelphia: W. B. Saunders.

Benner, P., & Wrubel, J. (1989). *The primacy of caring.* Menlo Park, CA: Addison-Wesley.

Bronowski, J. (1959). The values of science. In A. H. Maslow (Ed.), *New knowledge in human values* (pp. 52–64). South Bend, IN: Regnery/Gateway.

Carper, B. A. (1979). The ethics of caring. *Advances in Nursing Science, 2*, 11–19.

Fine, M. (1985). Reflections on a feminist psychology of women: Paradoxes and prospects. *Psychology of Women Quarterly, 9*, 167–183.

Fry, S. T. (1981). Accountability in research: The relationship of scientific and humanistic values. *Advances in Nursing Science, 4*, 1–13.

Gilligan, C. (1982). *In a different voice.* Cambridge: Harvard University Press.

Griffin, A. (1980). Philosophy and nursing. *Journal of Advanced Nursing, 5*, 261–271.

Grossinger, R. (1985). *Planet medicine: From stone age shamanism to post-industrial healing.* Berkeley: North Atlantic Books.

Harding, S. (1986). *The science question in feminism.* Ithaca, NY: Cornell University Press.

Keller, E. F. (1985). *Reflections on gender and science.* New Haven: Yale University Press.

Leininger, M. (1978). The phenomenon of caring: Importance, research questions and theoretical considerations. In *Caring: An essential human need: Proceedings of the three national caring conferences*. Thorofare, NJ: Slack.

LeShan, L., & Margenau, H. (1982). Structures of reality: Domains and realms. In *Einstein's space and Van Gogh's sky* (pp. 23–38). New York: Macmillan.

Levine, M. (1977, May). Nursing ethics and the ethical nurse. *American Journal of Nursing*, 845–849.

MacPherson, K. I. (1983, January). Feminist methods: A new paradigm for nursing research. *Advances in Nursing Science*, 17–25.

McBride, A. B., & McBride, W. L. (1982). Theoretical underpinnings for women's health. *Women & Health, 6*, 37–53.

Munhall, P. (1982). Nursing philosophy and nursing research: In apposition or opposition? *Nursing Research, 31*, 176–177.

Poslusny, S. (1989). Feminist friendship: Isabel Hampton Robb, Lavinia Lloyd Dock, and Adelaide Nutting. *Image, 21*(2), 64–68.

Robb, I. H. (1920). *Nursing ethics: For hospital and private use*. Cleveland: Koeckert, (Originally published in 1900).

Silva, M. (1977). Philosophy, science, theory: Interrelationships and implications for nursing research. *Image, 9*, 59–63.

Silva, M. C., & Rothbart, D. (1983). An analysis of changing trends in philosophies of science on nursing theory development and testing. *Advances in Nursing Science, 5*(1), 1–13.

Thompson, J. L. (1987). Critical scholarship: The critique of domination in nursing. *Advances in Nursing Science, 10*, 27–38.

Watson, J. (1981, July). Nursing's scientific quest. *Nursing Outlook*, 413–416.

15

Caring for Ourselves

Peggy Keen

As nursing continues to explore caring as a central focus for practice, it is important also to examine how nurses exhibit caring, or often lack of caring toward each other. It is crucial, however, to approach the examination of how we are caring or uncaring toward each other with the certainty that we have the power to change this. If we are unable to care first for ourselves as individuals, and then for our nursing colleagues, the caring that we give to our patients is not as good as it could be.

The talk that I will give was initially developed for a group of middle management nurses in a large public hospital in Atlanta. Unfortunately, I can only provide a brief glimpse of this previous effort, which was composed in a participatory manner. Although I've only had the opportunity to speak to this one group so far, my goal is to talk with as many nurses as possible about the process and importance of caring for each other. I also hope, by sharing my research, to inspire some of you to do a similar presentation to your nursing colleagues when you get home.

The idea that nurses should first focus on caring for each other is not new. In 1980, Ashley wrote that nursing would not accomplish it's goals of caring for others until we begin to make " . . . meaningful connections with the lives of other nurses and women, establishing a community of shared caring" (p. 21). She asserted that if nurses would begin to care for other nurses, the profession would have more than enough power necessary for positively shaping it's destiny.

We know what much of the current reality is like. Even if it is not our individual experience, we recognize that nurses generally are perceived as a fragmented group, where individuals are often isolated from one another. Nurses are not seen as having much solidarity. Often it seems like nurses don't move forward because of spending so much time and energy fighting each other. In fact, we frequently seem to devalue ourselves and each other (Ashley, 1980). But rather than accept the situation, it's critical to begin to look at how we got here in the first place.

I believe that we have gotten to a predominantly non-caring stance toward each other because nurses, due to who we are (primarily women) and what we do (undervalued work), are an *oppressed* group. Of course, oppression is a continuum. Obviously the oppression of American nurses is not comparable to the level of oppression experienced by a black person in South Africa or by women in certain third world countries who can be killed for not obeying their husbands. But it is clear that as a woman and as a nurse, I don't have all of the freedoms and power accorded to an educated, rich, white male in American society. It is also very clear that value accorded to work traditionally done by men has been, and still is, higher than work traditionally done by women. I won't try to tell you that I've experienced every single aspect or form of oppression, or convince you that you have either. I am also not here to accuse you individually of being uncaring toward your nursing colleagues. But I do believe that oppression directed at women and at the nursing profession by more powerful groups in the medical care/illness oriented system is the major reason that nurses, as a group, generally treat each other badly. Until we look carefully at how powerful groups have behaved toward us, and how their oppressive actions may have shaped our non-caring behaviors toward each other, we won't be able to make any positive changes (Freire, 1968).

As an aside, I've found that using the word *oppression* usually elicits strong reactions from people. The most common reaction is a look of acute discomfort complete with averted eyes and shifting around. This reaction intuitively feels like my words are being categorized as some sort of social fau paux; almost like using the word *feminist*. Another common reaction is that surely I'm overstating the case—things just can't be all that bad. I've also been told that everyone is oppressed in some way, and that oppression is too simple of a concept for the explanation of complex problems.

In my initial presentation, it was important to spend time defusing patriarchal notions about oppression. Since I don't need to do this in a self-selected feminist audience, we can move along to a quick review of a framework of characteristics of oppressor and oppressed behaviors.

This framework was initially developed by Andrianne Roy (1987), and is based on Pablo Freire's (1968) study of oppressed groups in Brazil. The framework was later collectively revised by Chinn, Wheeler, and Roy (1988) as a theoretical framework for an exploratory study of friendship among women nurses.

First, let's examine some characteristics of oppressors. These characteristics include:

—Oppressors operate from an ethic and consciousness of self-interest.

—Oppressors prescribe and define a "reality" for all to serve their interests (in the medical care delivery system we might think of this interest as maximum profit, and a reality that values curing over caring).

—Oppressors exploit and manipulate people for their own purposes.

—In order to do all of the previous three things, oppressors fail to recognize other beings as fully human.

There are certain conditions that ensure the continued domination of one group over another. These conditions include:

—Maintaining unequal educational opportunities between and among classes.

—Circumstances that assure divisions among the oppressed, e.g., the periodic granting of small favors.

—Enticement of members of the oppressed group to serve as tokens on behalf of the interests of the oppressor.

Oppression certainly does not occur in a vacuum. Chinn, Wheeler, and Roy (1988) maintained that oppression is only sustained by complementarity between groups—the dominant group can only exploit when the less powerful group is vulnerable to oppressive actions. As dominant groups bring pressure to bear on less powerful groups, the less powerful or oppressed groups cooperate in the oppression by beginning to exhibit certain characteristics.

According to Freire, cooperative behaviors of an oppressed group include:

—Beginning to internalize the consciousness of the oppressor, denying the self.

—Beginning to think and behave according to the prescriptions of the oppressor.

—Acting in ways that are not authentic.

All of the characteristics just mentioned facilitate the exploitation and manipulation of the oppressed group by the more powerful oppressor. The characteristics also further contribute to barriers to breaking free from oppression. Further, the oppressed group begins to:

> Deeply internalize the idea that the oppressor must be right by virtue of the imbalance of power.
>
> Fear freedom and begin to view themselves as incapable of taking risks.
>
> Have little or no desire to affiliate themselves with a powerless group.
>
> Exhibit a tendency to join with the oppressors and become suboppressors, so that they can also have power in the dominant system. (Chinn, Wheeler, & Roy, 1988)

This construct of oppression helped me to recognize some of the forces that have been influencing women and nurses as individuals, and which have been undermining the profession as a whole. However, for my own understanding of the phenomenon of oppression, I needed to go further and look at some tangible ways in which nurses might produce and reproduce oppressive divisive dynamics that create uncaring behaviors toward each other.

Building on the work of Ashley (1976, 1980), Torres (1981), Roberts (1983), and Roy (1987), I organized an oppression checklist, "Is Your Oppression Showing?" Some of the questions on the checklist had been raised by the women I just mentioned while others came from my own experience with oppressive "traps"; traps which were usually only recognized as I was crawling out of them. I devised this checklist not as a way of judging our behavior, but as a way to understand the behavior. The intent of the checklist is also to provide a way for nurses to recognize and talk about their own experiences.

Remember that oppressor groups continually send messages downward that prescribe and define reality—that tell us what's good or bad. The oppressed group begins to internalize the values and consciousness of the oppressor. This first set of "have you ever" questions reflects what I call "overt messages from the patriarchy"—things we are told, which we begin to believe, and in turn begin to say about ourselves.

Values/Consciousness of the Oppressor - Denying Self
Have you ever???

. . . referred to females (over the age of 18) as girls?

. . . said "it's really hard to work with a bunch of women"?

. . . believed that it is impossible, or at least very difficult, for women to reach a consensus?

. . . said or felt that most of your friends were men . . . or you just can't trust women/women are so catty/women are such back stabbers?

. . . said you always prefer a male boss over a female one?

. . . believed that men have more natural leadership ability than women?

. . . taken a man's medical complaint more seriously than a woman's (in a similar situation)?

. . . tried especially hard to be objective, logical, and unemotional in your daily worklife?

. . . gotten more frequently rewarded by others (not patients) for the performance of technological tasks than for meeting the psychosocial needs of patients?

. . . felt that the part of nursing that you enjoy doing the most is considered the least important?

Subtle messages in the above category include such things as "men are smarter, more organized, more rational, better leaders, and it's the natural order of things for them to be IN CHARGE" . . . you know the ones. These messages are internalized and result in negative comments about women in ways which reveal a denial of self. Comments of this type perpetuate negative judgements about the way women are, and serve to entrench destructive stereotypes. Because of these negative messages, women distance themselves from themselves—they disconnect from the self that is female.

For me, one of the most graphic examples of the behavior of denying self presented itself on an elevator. I was riding down to the ground floor, and a woman got on about half-way down. Some time after the door closed she suddenly turned to me and with a great deal of passion said "don't you just hate to work with a bunch of women?" Before I could fully comprehend or react to what she said, the door opened and she got off. I was so astounded that I missed my floor—I remember thinking "just who or what did I look like to her?" (I even had a skirt on that day!) But there are many other ways in which negative, patriarchal ideas about women are reproduced. I've listed some others in the first category given.

When we continually hear messages from both men and women that tell us we are second class citizens, this understandably undermines our self-esteem.

We act in ways which are painfully self-depreciating and debasing. Some of these ways are listed in the next category.

Behaviors prescribed by the Oppressor-Issues of Self-Esteem Have you ever???

. . . prefaced statements with phrases such as "I know this is a really stupid question"/"I'm sure I don't really understand this but . . . ?"

. . . found it difficult to accept compliments—instead of saying thank you, you respond with phrases such as . . . "it really wasn't anything" . . . "it wasn't hard, anybody could have done it?"

. . . felt or said that you were "unworthy" of an honor or award?

. . . constantly compared yourself with others (Jane is skinnier, nicer, a better speaker)?

. . . thought that if a nurse has more education than you: (a) she must know more than you do and you feel inferior or (b) she might have a higher degree but probably is less capable of doing less actual hands on nursing, and you feel superior?

. . . taken time for yourself just to relax, reflect, or do something nice for yourself?

For example, statements prefaced with "I know this is stupid, I really don't deserve this," saying and feeling we're unworthy of honors or awards are evidence of lack of self-esteem. If we're constantly told we are unworthy, we begin to believe and express feelings of unworthiness.

Also included in this category is the detrimental idea that women must constantly compete with each other. We learn, as children, to compete for men, but the behavior seems to persist, even after we get one, or decide we don't want one. Men also get to dictate standards of beauty and other "desirable" attributes, and then rank women in a hierarchy according to how many of these artificial attributes we possess.

Finally, you can check your personal level of self-esteem with the last question because when you feel as if you have worth, you *do* spend some time caring for yourself. It may not be much time, but it is a conscious effort. As Elizabeth Cady Stanton said "to develop our real selves, we need time alone for thought and meditation. To always be giving out and never pumping in, the well runs dry too soon" (p. 573).

Because we are told that we are worthless, and because we start to feel that way, we ignore internal messages—messages from the heart that reflect how we want to be, how we know we could and should be. We give up our ability to act in authentic, or real ways. A few of the ways in which unauthentic behaviors are manifested are listed in the next category.

Authenticity
Have you ever???

. . . believed very strongly that something you were told to do was wrong, but acquiesced in order not to "rock the boat"?

. . . changed your "story" according to the audience? (For example, in a meeting with nursing administrators, you verbally endorse a plan, offering no negative comments. Then, when describing the plan to other nurses, you present only your frustrations with the plan.)

. . . complained about a problem to your fellow nurses but did nothing to confront the person you believe is causing the problem?

. . . believed that it is never appropriate for nurses (or women) to get angry?

A common behavior I've observed among nurses—we remain outwardly complacent even when something is bothering us so that we aren't labeled troublemakers or, God forbid, "unladylike." This denial of feelings is obviously related to job burnout.

All behaviors prescribed by the oppressor that contribute to denial of self, low self-esteem, and the inability to act authentically make exploitation easier. The needs of the oppressor are satisfied, while the needs of the less powerful group are ignored. In the next category, I've listed several examples of exploitation.

Exploitation/Unmet Personal Needs
Have you ever???

. . . allowed yourself to be addressed in a familiar way by someone while feeling compelled (or being required) to address that person in a more formal way (i.e., "Good morning Jane" . . . . "Good morning Dr. Smith")?

. . . found yourself playing the nurse-doctor game where your significant recommendations must be presented in such a manner as to make the action appear to be initiated by the physician?

. . . left work feeling frustrated about an incident that you were
involved in where policy prohibited you from implementing the
right course of action?

. . . encountered a situation where, when pressure for change has
come from nurses, you were offered token gestures of appease-
ment but the real problem was not addressed or changed?

Having their own efforts go unrecognized, or having their efforts credited
to medicine, is one example of exploitation that many nurses talk about having
experienced. The final question in this section is an example of how needs of
an oppressed group are not addressed, but uprisings are successfully quelled
(we probably all have classic examples of this occurring).

Remember that the behavior of the oppressed group itself can further
create barriers to freedom or liberation. The next category of behaviors on the
checklist are ways in which nurses conform to oppressor ideals or demonstrate that they don't particularly want to be associated with other nurses.

Conforming to Oppressor Ideals to Achieve Power
Have you ever???

. . . preferred to be associated with professional groups other
than nursing (i.e., AHA as opposed to ANA)?

. . . preferred alliance with specialty organizations instead of
groups representing general nursing? (The nurse practitioners have
it so much more together than those "Other" nurses!)

. . . thought that your career would benefit more from doing a
presentation for a national medical group (i.e., ACOG) than for
a national nursing group (i.e., NAACOG)?

. . . felt (good/superior/vindicated/proud) when a physician told
you . . . "I really trust/respect/listen to you, you're different
from most nurses"?

. . . considered it a great compliment when told "you're so smart,
you should have gone to medical school"?

. . . at work, dressed in a way that more closely resembled medicine
than nursing?

The above questions represent ways in which nurses either demean nursing or emulate medicine in order to identify with the more powerful group.
As a result, nurses choose to be more closely associated with other professional groups, or get involved only in specialty nursing organizations and

remain fragmented instead of belonging to both a mainstream nursing group and a group that meets particular nursing needs. This is one reason why we may like it when people tell us we're different from most nurses. Considering it a great compliment when told that "you're so smart you should have gone to medical school" is a particularly pervasive example of this type of behavior.

The last category is also worthy of in-depth consideration. Isn't it interesting to think about how, as nurses ascend their professional hierarchy, nurses begin to dress more like physicians (i.e., street clothes and lab coats instead of uniforms)? Although uniforms are somewhat oppressive, that is a subject for another discussion. However, the process of identification with a group that is perceived to have more power is clear enough.

Oppressed people who ardently buy into the system become tokens of the system. They acquire power (but never full power), and begin to act as suboppressors. Some of these behaviors are reflected by the questions in the next category.

Marginality
Have you ever???

. . . felt that nurses in power positions "over you" have more loyalty to physicians/administrators than they do to nursing?

. . . compromised beliefs in order to get promoted/make more money?

. . . hesitated to tell someone that you've just met at a party that you're a nurse?

. . . valued a compliment more highly when it came from a medical colleague than when it came from a nursing colleague?

. . . resisted change because you feel more comfortable in a familiar environment or because you believe you have superior knowledge (or power) related to the current way in which things are being done?

If you've had the feeling that nurses have more loyalty to medicine or to the hospital administration than they do to nursing, you've probably been right. Rewards provided by an oppressive system are very effective in the creation and maintenance of token suboppressors.

Another example of marginality, and conformity to a system which doesn't value nursing can occur when a nurse obtains another title and stops identifying him or herself as a nurse. I have a nursing friend who, when she started working for a large government health agency that will remain nameless (even though it is located in Atlanta), was told that she could not list her RN credentials on her business card. The rationale for this omission was that physicians she had to consult within her job would not listen to what she was saying if they knew she was a nurse. She really wanted the position, and is now called a medical epidemiologist. She is truly one of nursing's brightest and best, and she now works in a system that will not recognize her as a nurse.

The final category, horizontal violence, lists some examples of how a nurse's generally low sense of self-esteem is reflected in overtly uncaring behaviors directed toward other nurses.

Horizontal Violence/Self-Hatred
Have you ever???

. . . said that we (nurses) are our own worst enemy?

. . . after having a terrible day, reflect your frustrations toward other nurses more frequently than physicians?

. . . found yourself more frequently making comments (either positive or negative ones) about other nurses rather than to the other nurses that were the focus of your comments?

. . . experienced more jealousy/envy over the success of a female colleague than over the success of a male colleague?

. . . gotten angry at the profession of nursing over something that was really the "fault" of others?

. . . been described, or thought of yourself as controlling or rigid?

. . . felt that your past educational or job experiences were supervised by people who were controlling or rigid?

After all, if I'm not personally valuable, then you, also a nurse, must not be valuable or worthy of my respect either. We've all seen, and I know I've frequently participated in horizontal violence—I get yelled at inappropriately by a physician or administrator, and in turn, snap at another nurse, or better yet, holler at the nursing assistant who of course has less power than I do, who may in turn take it out on the patient, typically the least powerful of all.

In this category, the statement that "nurses are our own worst enemy" is my least favorite although it does identify a certain truth. As used, this statement provides reason to the charge that nursing is a hopeless profession that will never change; no doubt, a bad case of blaming the victim.

Also included in this category are behaviors which involve *talking about* other people rather than *to* other people. Interactions of this type present a major barrier to caring for each other. If nurses never communicate directly with each other, nurses will never connect on a personal level, and caring cannot occur.

The last two questions in this section are concerned with rigid, controlling behaviors. While these may not obviously exhibit horizontal violence, Freire (1968) maintained that the characteristics of being rigid or controlling come not only from low self-esteem and marginality, but also from hatred of your own kind.

Finally, the last question on the checklist asks whether you believe that nursing does not have the ability to change. The belief that people are truly powerless to change a situation is an ultimate symptom of oppression.

As stated earlier, the purpose of using the framework of oppression and the provided checklist was not to further reify uncaring nurse-to-nurse behaviors. Rather, the purpose was to discuss perhaps unconscious behaviors so that nurses can examine them with greater clarity and, hopefully, begin to change uncaring behaviors. As Freire (1968) asserted, it is necessary to unveil the world of oppression in order to transform it.

At first glance, it may appear that change is a difficult, if not impossible project. After all, nurses have endured and adapted to such a long history of being oppressed. In addition, the oppressive system is complex and appears exceptionally powerful. Nonetheless, I believe that changing is as easy as *stopping*—refusing to act like an oppressed group and ceasing, as Gray (1987) said, to dance with the dominator. We must put away our dancing pumps (mine are worn down anyway!) forevermore.

Change won't come all at once—even though it probably could if we all quit dancing at the same time. But it can happen. Change comes with vowing to always watch out for the oppressive traps on the checklist. It involves taking a solemn oath that the words "nursing is its own worst enemy" will never again pass our lips, unless it's said among ourselves as we work to change our way of being nurses. Change happens when we begin to recognize that when we interact with one another from a place of frail ego, self-hatred, or competition, the oppressor is again "having his way with us."

It's as easy as deciding, here and now, in this room, that we will direct energy toward caring for ourselves and each other. It begins with knowing, that as women and as nurses, that we contribute something of value to the world, that caring and curing are complimentary processes, and that one should not be valued more than the other. Change also involves recognizing that since individually we are wonderful, strong, caring people, the colleagues that share this outstanding profession must be valuable and worthy of our caring too.

Because changing consciousness facilitates action (Starhawk, 1982), changing our consciousness can change our reality. Starhawk maintained "When we take action, we reclaim our content, our sense of our own authority and value.

We reclaim our power—not the ability to dominate another, but the power of consciousness immanent within us—the power to heal, to change, to create. Whenever we love (or show caring for one another) we create community" (p. 182).

Glendinning (1982) noted that patriarchy typically insists that power lies outside the individual and oppressed individuals often cease to believe in their own inner power, if they've even recognized it was there to begin with. But it's there—it's just a matter of reclaiming this power.

Power to care for ourselves and for other nurses is created through our thoughts and feelings. First, we must grant power to ourselves, and appropriate our individual internal power. Then the discovery and empowerment of self increasingly leads to the discovery of, and connection with, others. The power to care will increase in proportion to our belief in the necessity of caring for ourselves and each other, and to the extent to which this belief is communicated to nurses both within this room and beyond it.

Below are specific recommendations about actions that can bring our new "caring for each other consciousness" into reality. Although these may sound simple, they are a beginning effort to create a different reality of caring for ourselves and each other.

1. Take time every day to be alone for some self-to-self communication. The time doesn't have to be long, and in fact doesn't always even have to physically be there. But the intention, the thought that it is necessary to do something to care for yourself should be a conscious and reinforcing presence.

2. Make it a point, at least once a day, to say something positive or nurturing to a nursing colleague. It can't be something you make up—it has to be something you feel. It's not as if the people we work with don't ever do wonderful things—they do them constantly. Trying this once a day can change the focus from being neutral or more ready to find something negative, to a focus of actively searching for something positive. Do not become embarrassed when people begin to call you Pollyanna. I'm convinced that this behavior will catch on.

3. Tell Hero stories. I first heard this recommendation from Mary Mallison (1987), who pointed out that we don't do enough of sharing of our proud moments. Telling hero stories is a way to help us celebrate nurses and nursing. Tell hero stories to your friends outside of nursing, to your family, to your students, to the media, and of course to other nurses.

If you don't know many hero stories, meet for a beer and swap some around. It's always beneficial to increase your repertoire.

4. Seek mentors or be mentors for other nurses. It's a way of actively committing the sharing of yourself in a very personal way with the profession.

5. Make chances to envision how nursing can be—in this case, how we want to care for ourselves and each other. Imagine a new world, a new way of being and acting at every opportunity. Copper (1982) contended that by visualizing what we want in relation to each other, new patterns of interaction are given life. Women need new definitions of honor which emphasize the importance of noncompetitive interactions, reciprocity, and nurturance. Sharing, mutual validation, and emotional support are also needed to begin our healing process with each other. We do these things for other people. We just need to make it a priority to nurture ourselves and other nurses.

As an example of this envisioning process, my classmates at Georgia State University and I, guided by Dr. Patty Gray, created a Center for Nursing Research operated according to feminist principles. We envisioned the Center primarily as a place of *resourcement*, a word used by Mary Daly to describe a source of life and spirit. Our "Vision Beyond" (as we called it) was very detailed, but I'll share only a few of the highlights here. First, the Resourcement Center would house a rotating "core" group of visionary nurses, whose main purpose would be to inspire the profession to new heights, to organize nurses "in the trenches" and to help facilitate a network for the continuous flow of new ideas. It would have a place where any nurse could come to rest, and be nurtured, and go back out fully energized (child care provided of course!). If you couldn't come to the Center in person, you could call the Hotline—and never be put on hold.

A mission of the Center would be to recognize and further develop interconnectedness, and to continually work to eliminate separation and barriers between nurses, nurses and patients, and nurses and society. Of course, people at the Center would all have a copy of *Peace and Power, Guidelines for Feminist Process* by Wheeler and Chinn (1984) and would continually work together to remember the wisdom of Doing what we Know, as layers of patriarchal learning and conditioning are shed.

Not forgetting research, the structure for funding would be nonhierarchical, and qualitative research would be just as valuable as quantitative research.

The Center would demonstrate faith in many new researchers, and in vision-ary studies that could help to move us beyond the current system. Ideas for research would even be generated by patients, who will of course sit on the rotating funding board.

The telling and sharing of visions helps us to see possibilities and create change. I encourage you to use the power of your own imagination to create and nurture visions of nurses demonstrating increased caring for each other, and for anything else that needs changing in the profession.

Finally, make a continuous attempt to connect with your nursing past. Not only the collective nursing past, even though it's important to recognize the heroes and visionaries who have come before us, but your personal nursing past. Every time I am tempted to go and sell real estate instead of being a nurse, it helps me to recall that the neatest, most centered, most loving, caring, people that I know in the world are nurses. In my childhood, one woman showed me a different way of being. She was a nurse and I wanted to be like her, so I chose nursing as a career. In my adult life, women, mainly my nursing friends from school and work, have been there to help me through the hard times. They've also come together to create and share some of the best times in my life. Our network of caring remains strong, even though many of us now live all over the country and can't see each other very often. I don't think my friends and I are unique, even though stereotypes (those voices of the oppressor) continue to enforce the notion that women generally don't like each other.

Remember who has given you support and nurturance in your life, and I'll bet there will be at least a few nurses in the group. We need to take the caring connections with other nurses that we personally recall, and send that positive and loving energy that we have received outward in an ever widening circle so that, as energy meets energy, the caring energy will be powerful enough to encompass the entire profession.

To help with remembering, I would like to close with a short slide show of my own rememberings of times shared with nursing friends and from nursing programs where I've been a student or a teacher. These are my friends and my memories, but they could just as easily be yours. As you feel your memories, and focus on nurses caring for other nurses, I would like to leave you with some more wise words from Starhawk (1982) who said "against forces of destruction (such as oppression), we have only our human will and imagina-tion, our courage, our passion, our willingness (to care and to) love. The power that is in us is a *great*, if not INVINCIBLE power. It can hurt, but it can also heal. It can destroy, but it can also renew. And it is morning. And there is still time to choose" (p. 182).

REFERENCES

Ashley, J. (1973, October, 21). This I believe: About power in nursing. *Nursing Outlook*, 638–642.

Ashley, J. (1976). *Hospital, paternalism, and the role of the nurse.* New York: Teachers College Press.

Ashley, J. (1980, April). Power in structured misogyny: Implications for the politics of care. *Advances in Nursing Science, 2*(3), 3–21.

Chinn, P., Wheeler, C., & Roy, A. (1988). *Theoretical framework—exploratory study of friendship among women nurses.* Unpublished manuscript.

Copper, B. (1982). The voice of women's spirituality in futurism. In C. Spretnak (Ed.), *The politics of women's spirituality.* Garden City, NJ: Anchor Books, 497–509.

Daly, M. (1978). *Gyn/Ecology: The metaethics of radical feminism.* Boston: Beacon Press.

Dressel, P. (1987). Patriarchy and social welfare work. *Social Problems, 34*(3), 294–309.

DuBois, E., Kelly, G., Kennedy, E., Korsmeyer, C., & Robinson, L. (1985). Women's oppression: Understanding the dimensions. In *Feminist Scholarship.* Chicago: University of Illinois Press.

Freire, P. (1968). *Pedagogy of the oppressed.* New York: Seabury Press.

Frye, M. (1983). Oppression. In *The politics of reality: Essays in feminist theory.* Trumansburg, NY: Crossing Press.

Glendinning, C. (1982). The healing powers of women. In C. Spretnak (Ed.), *The politics of women's spirituality.* Garden City, NJ: Anchor Books, 280–293.

Gray, P. (1987). Presentation. Georgia State University.

Hartmann, H. (1976). Capitalism, patriarchy, and job segregation by sex. In M. Blaxall & B. Regan (Eds.), *Woman and the workplace: The implications of occupational segregation.* Chicago: University of Chicago Press, 137–169.

Mallision, M. (1987). Presentation to the Georgia Nurses' Association, Macon, Georgia.

Reverby, S. (1981). A caring dilemma: Womanhood and nursing in historical perspective. *Nursing Research, 36*(1), 5–10.

Rich, A. (1976). *Of woman born: Motherhood as experience and institution.* New York: W. W. Norton.

Roberts, S. (1983, July). Oppressed group behavior: Implications for nursing. *Advances in Nursing Science,* 21-30.

Roy, A. (1987). Come, unity . . . Creating a community in nursing. *Cassandra, 5*(2), 16-19.

Spretnak, C. (Ed.). (1982). *The politics of women's spirituality.* Garden City, NY: Anchor Press.

Starhawk (1982). Consciousness, politics, and magic. In C. Spretnak (Ed.), *The politics of women's spirituality.* Garden City, NJ: Anchor Books, 172-184.

Torres, G. (1981, March). The nursing education administrator: Accountable, vulnerable and oppressed. *Advances in Nursing Science,* 1-16.

Vance, C. (1979). Woman leaders: Modern day heroines or societal deviants? *Image, 11*(2), 37-41.

Wheeler, C., & Chinn, P. (1984). *Peace and power: A handbook of feminist process.* Buffalo, NY: Margaretdaughters.

16

Feminist Pedagogy: Nurturing the Ethical Ideal

Margaret A. Crowley

The use of case studies as a means for examining moral problems and ethical dilemmas in clinical practice has a tradition in nursing. I will continue this tradition by presenting a case study that enlarges the realm of discourse beyond the nurse-patient-physician-institution relationship to include the student and nurse educator.

This real life scenario features a nursing student and a nursing faculty member. Pseudonyms will be used—Maureen for the clinical instructor and Rebecca for the student. The student–teacher interaction and details of the context, which will aid in the analysis of this situation, are also presented.

THE SCENARIO

The baccalaureate nursing program that Maureen and Rebecca were affiliated with had devised an intensive practicum experience for students to take place in the final semester of the senior year. Students were placed in a clinical agency for 32–40 hours a week. Direct support to the students came from an onsite preceptor, a staff nurse within the institution. Maureen was the clinical faculty member from the university who visited the students in each agency on a weekly basis and conducted a weekly clinical seminar on campus.

There were three weeks remaining in the semester when Maureen arrived at the nursing conference room for the weekly clinical conference. She asked if anyone would like to begin by recounting any events from the previous week. Rebecca began:

> I was in the labor and delivery room this week and you won't believe what happened. There was a young, unmarried Spanish-speaking girl who was about to deliver. She was screaming and crying out in pain. Dr. Westerman, the obstetrician, was getting everything ready for the delivery when he just walked up to the head of the delivery table, didn't say anything and slapped her across the face twice. I guess I must have made some kind of a face like I was surprised or something because he looked at me and said: "Are you related to her?" and I said "No." So he said to me: "Well then, what's the face for?" Maureen interjected: "What happened then, Rebecca?" and Rebecca responded: "Oh, nothing really. He just went about delivering the baby."

In recounting this incident, Maureen was stunned by the student's response. She explained:

> I felt that her response, and that of the other students present, was nothing more than: "Isn't this an interesting story?" I asked Rebecca how the staff nurses in attendance had responded. She stated that "They didn't do anything." The staff told her: "That's just the way Dr. Westerman is." I asked next: "Is there anything you feel that you need to do?" I sensed that Rebecca was getting a little nervous now. She seemed to know that she was responding to me the wrong way if she stated that she felt no responsibility to do anything. She started to do what I call backpedalling: "But he didn't really hit her that hard. And, she really was hysterical." I think she really knew that she had made a mistake now when I responded: "REBECCA, I don't care if all he did was raise his hand to her. What he did was WRONG." I told her that I wanted her to think the situation over during the weekend and I would meet with her at the hospital on Monday to find out what she had decided to do. I told her that she did not have to finish out the final three weeks of the practicum, that she had met the objectives of the course already. I also said that I would go with her to do whatever she felt needed to be done. I stated: "If you decide not to report this incident, I shall have to. Now that I know about this situation, I have an obligation to do something."

Maureen continued:

> I met with her on Monday and she said that she wanted to talk with the staff herself and tell them that she was going to write up an incident report. Later, I found out that she told the staff that I was making her write the incident report. She told them that I had found out about the incident by reading her weekly journal. I stated that the report should indicate that a copy would go to the dean of the nursing program. I wanted the staff to know that this incident was being reported beyond the institution. Rebecca's original report stated in effect that: "The patient was hysterical and screaming uncontrollably. In an effort to calm her down, Dr. Westerman slapped her on the face." I was really becoming exasperated with Rebecca at this point. It seemed to me that she was doing everything that she could do to get out of this situation. "Just give me the facts, Rebecca! No editorializing!" I told her as I read the report. She rewrote it until I found it to be acceptable.
>
> The following week in clinical seminar, the incident came up again briefly in our discussion. I was again stunned when the students stated that they probably would have responded the way Rebecca had—that they would choose to do nothing. "After all, we're only students" was the overriding theme that I gleaned from their comments. And, my response, now coming from a sense of complete frustration was: "And someday, you'll only be a staff nurse, or you'll only be a part-time nurse, or you'll only be an agency nurse!"
>
> Rebecca met with me for one last conference during the final week of the practicum. She had decided to stay on the unit to finish out the semester. She could barely speak to me at this point. I knew that anything that I had to say now would be useless.

Maureen's final comments to me were:

> The whole incident left me terribly depressed. I felt that I, that we as nursing faculty, were failing if this was how our students were behaving as they entered the world of work. I have asked students in subsequent years how they would have responded given this situation and many of them have said the same thing: "I probably would have chosen to do nothing." One student recently stated: "It's very important for the staff to like you during the practicum. It's important to do things the way they do them."

ANALYSIS

This situation can be analyzed from two vantage points. First, Maureen's response to the situation within the context of who she is as a nurse educator will be explored. What follows is a reconstruction of this incident keeping in mind that Maureen's primary goal as a teacher should be what Noddings (1984) refers to as "nurturance of the ethical ideal" within the student (p. 173).

Before beginning, this author must share her own position in this matter as a feminist:

I felt as troubled as my colleague did for some of the same and also perhaps for some different reasons. I too was shocked by the incident. Here was one more example of the abuse of particularly vulnerable, defenseless, and power-less women by physicians. And, nurses were still, in a sense, normalizing this kind of behavior in the orientation of new nurses into the system by saying, in essence: "This is Dr. Jones. He induces all of his patients with Pitocin. This is Dr. Westerman. He hits his patients sometimes."

I admired my colleague for doing what was right. Here was a woman who was not willing to accept the status quo. The more Maureen and I discussed this situation, however, the more dissatisfied we became. If Maureen was right and Rebecca was wrong, had Rebecca learned anything from this situation? Would Rebecca go on to behave differently in the future? We reluctantly admitted that she probably would not. In fact, we believed that she would instead keep such incidents to herself. We both felt more and more distance from our students. Who were these women who saw the world so differently from us?

The Teacher's Response

Pence (1987) examined nursing ethics literature and classified approaches to nursing ethics in three ways:

1. The application of the major consequentialist and deontological theories to ethical issues.

2. The use of traditional moral principles and ideals to guide discussion of moral problems—(e.g., the principle of fidelity or the principle of autonomy).

3. The philosophical foundations approach where ". . . ethical issues are dealt with from the perspective of a philosophical conception of the nature of nursing" (p. 7).

I contend that Maureen's response was based in part on the use of traditional moral principles and ideals and the philosophical foundations approach. Furthermore, I hope to demonstrate that neither of these approaches is adequate as a pedagogical model for nurturing the ethical ideal in the student. This is not to suggest that these approaches do not serve as useful models for moral education. But as pedagogical models, they must be preceded by an ethics of care, an ethic that is foundational to all student–teacher interactions.

Moral Principles Approach

Pence (1987) explains that with the moral principles approach, exemplified in the now classic work of Beauchamp and Childress (1983), moral principles rooted in moral theory are the basis for ethical action. These principles serve as the justification for moral action. In this case, Maureen's response to Rebecca appears to be grounded in the ethical principle of non-maleficence ("What he did was harmful.") Maureen viewed Rebecca as guilty of violating the same principle by association. I might add, however, that Maureen never articulated her moral perspective clearly to either me or the student. Hersh, Paolitto, and Reiner (1979) note that in situations in which the teacher does not go beyond an expression of value to the explication of a specific moral principle, the complexity of moral education is avoided. The teacher solves the ethical problem through the use of positional power rather than through clear exploration of the moral perspectives underlying the teacher's or the student's position.

Veatch and Fry (1987) note that both medicine and nursing ethics have a tradition of invoking the principle of producing good (beneficence) and avoiding harm (non-maleficence). The principle is stated specifically in the Hippocratic Oath, the Florence Nightingale Pledge (Kalisch & Kalisch, 1986), and the ANA Code for Nurses (American Nurses' Association, 1985). A balance must often be struck between doing good and avoiding harm. Veatch and Fry point out that some ethicists believe that the charge to do no harm is a weightier responsibility than to do good. In fact, Maureen felt that no good at all could possibly have resulted from the physicians actions.

Sara Hoagland (1986), a feminist philosopher, views the moral principles approach as consistent with the Anglo-European tradition in philosophy, a tradition in which the first goal is to establish moral agency. One essentially tries to determine if an individual is morally accountable for his or her actions. The individual is judged not accountable only if he or she could not have done otherwise, if their actions were somehow determined "by a benevolent god or an indifferent mechanistic universe" (p. 74). Hoagland argues that this conception of moral agency is inadequate for actually dealing with the complex environments where nurses function. She contends that this view of moral agency

does not take into account what moral accountability would mean under conditions of oppression.

It may be useful at this juncture to examine the conditions under which the
student was operating. Yarling and McElmurray (1986) and Pitts (1985) provide
insights into the socialization process that occurs during the course of nursing
education. They describe a covert curriculum operating in insidious ways to
undermine the explicit educational processes. Yarling and McElmurray write:

> "Oh no," you say, "that can't be. Student nurses today are taught
> that nursing requires patient advocacy, that patient care comes first."
> Yes, that is what they are taught verbally and overtly; but in a
> thousand nonverbal and covert ways, they are taught by clinical
> example the limits of advocacy. They learn quickly by observing
> others, how to interpret the verbal message in terms of "what nurses
> do" and "what nurses do not do." They learn that their commitment
> to patients must be carefully contained. (p. 67)

A number of authors (Yarling & McElmurray, 1986; Roberts, 1983;
Thompson, 1987) have described the nature of the oppression undermining
the position of nurses within the health care subculture. It is in this context of
clinical practice that new practitioners are socialized in ". . . as powerful and
thorough . . . [a way as] . . . the verbal and ideological socialization in the
education context" (Yarling & McElmurray, p. 67).

Once moral agency is determined, the next step, according to Hoagland
(1986, 1987), is the examination of excuses and then the assignment of praise or
blame. The two general categories of excuses identified by Aristotle (1976) are
ignorance and constraint or physical restraint. Once excuses are found to be
inadequate and unacceptable, we are then called upon to sit in judgment of the
other, to assign praise for heroism or blame for failure to act according to
the appropriate principle. Again, Hoagland finds this process lacking in the
necessary complexity needed for dealing with moral agency under conditions of
oppression. By assigning praise or blame under conditions of oppression,
Hoagland notes, we run the risk of either blaming the victim—holding the
individual responsible for everything that happens to him or her, or the converse—victimism—assuming that the individual is a total victim who cannot be
held responsible for making choices.

In this scenario, Maureen has determined that both the physician and
Rebecca are morally accountable. Rebecca's accountability relates to her failure to take action in response to the situation.

Noddings (1984) warns, "We may become dangerously self-righteous when
we perceive ourselves as holding a precious principle not held by the other. The

other may then be devalued and treated 'differently'" (p. 5). Indeed, I think we have witnessed this assessment of "difference" between nursing faculty and students. I have heard quoted at a number of recent nursing conferences the results of a study conducted with graduating high school students approximately 20 years ago and now redone with today's graduates for purposes of comparison. While we, the high school students of 20 years ago, hoped to save the world, all they, the high school students of today, want to do is to make a great deal of money. Beliefs such as these set nursing educators apart from their students and allow the educators to stand in judgment of the students and to find their behavior wanting.

Philosophical Foundations Approach

"On this approach," Pence (1987) writes, ". . . fundamental issues in nursing ethics stem from the views one holds about the nature and function of nursing" (p. 9). The focus now becomes the profession of nursing and the various "role[s] function[s] and professional obligations" (p. 9) that are seen as fulfilling the ideal of nursing. Exploring the role of the nurse as patient advocate has been the central focus of the work done in this area. This signals a significant departure from the traditional view of nursing. Now the nurse is obligated first to be loyal to the patient or client rather than the physician or institution. Similar to the moral principles approach, the philosophical foundations approach seeks to establish moral accountability. In this instance, moral accountability is based on the enactment of a specific nursing role.

I contend that Maureen had a vision of the kind of role a nurse should play given this type of situation. In fact, I would hypothesize that many nursing faculty go into teaching out of a failure to enact their idealized vision of a nursing role and that nursing faculty often have a clearly articulated conception of the ideal roles for nurses. This vision of specific roles for nurses is problematic when used as a model for resolving ethical issues and dilemmas with students. The enactment of a prescribed role allows nurses to avoid making choices; the choices have already been made. Hoagland (1986) alludes to de Beauvoir's notion of ready-made values when she writes: ". . . the 'serious man' pretends value is ready-made and hides behind a role. He is not a person but a father. As a result, he claims he is compelled to do certain things. (It is his duty) . . . He pretends the value he chooses is outside him and that he is subordinating himself to it" (p. 79). Indeed, the nursing students alluded to these predetermined choices when they protested—"But we're only nursing students"—as a defense for their lack of response. Somehow they saw the invisible armour of that student role as protection and justification for their lack of moral accountability in this situation.

The other problematic issue with regard to role is that the faculty–student relationship may become much like the parent–child relationship when the teacher has a richly detailed vision of the nurse. The nursing faculty are in danger of having a somewhat different relationship with their students than other faculty members have. For example, an English professor may teach hundreds of students in a given year and among these, there may be only one student who knows today that he or she wishes to pursue the same career as the professor. By contrast, as nursing faculty, we are in a sense reproducing ourselves. It is much harder for nursing educators to separate themselves from their students because they prepare the students to replace them. When a student is confronted with an ethical dilemma, the nursing educator wants him or her to do what the educator would do or should have done. And these expectations are communicated to the student either overtly or covertly. Noddings (1984) cautions against this relationship in which the parent (or teacher) "lives for" the child (or student). According to Noddings, there is often subtle pressure on the student to do what the teacher wishes he or she might have done. In this case, Rebecca appears to be responding in a way many educators are familiar with. She has tried to "psych out" her teacher in order to determine the correct course of action.

Rich (1976) describes the effects of powerlessness (in this instance, the powerlessness of a student involved in a clearly hierarchical student–teacher relationship) on the psyche of the powerless. She writes:

> Powerlessness can lead to lassitude, self-negation, guilt, and depression; it can also generate a kind of psychological keenness, a shrewdness, an alert and practiced observation of the oppressor — "psyching out" developed into a survival tool. (p. 65)

Pence (1987) points to the now classic work of Yarling and McElmurray (1986) as yet another example of the philosophical foundations approach. In this article, the argument is made that ". . . nurses are often not free to be moral" (p. 63). Because their acts are often the result of forced choices, the authors conclude attention must be focused on the larger social agenda and institutional constraints to moral action must be addressed. Hoagland (1986), on the other hand, does not deny that there are conditions of oppression that force nurses into choices. But she adds that she is:

> . . . not focusing on them, since oppressors are already in the business of undermining other's moral agency and we can't count on them to cease once the folly of their ways has been pointed out (over and over I might add). The oppressed still go on under oppression and

make choices even when coerced and exploited. To conclude simply that [in the case of Rebecca, she isn't] to blame for choices because [she is] oppressed isn't helpful. For [she] still [has] to go on with [her life] and make further choices as do all under oppression. (p. 86)

If educators focus exclusively on the larger social agenda for ethical practice rather than the complex issues that must be dealt with in daily practice, they serve to further distance themselves from students rather than becoming engaged in the lived, caring encounter of the student and the patient. Educators should be wary of their ideologies becoming what this author calls *idiolotries* that serve to set them above their students in an abstract world of isms. In this instance, Maureen seems to have lost sight of the experiences of both the young woman in labor and the student by focusing primarily on ethical principles and philosophical foundations.

An Ethics of Care

According to Hoagland (1987), the process that Maureen was engaged in, the process of judging, of ". . . pointing the blaming finger, is not likely to change long time patterns" (p. 26). She adds further: ". . . a primary focus on praise and blame keeps our attention exclusively on ourselves, or alternatively on the bad person and not on the interactive nature of the situation . . ." (p. 27).

Recasting this scenario with an ethics of care as the pedagogic model changes the focus to the interdependent nature of peoples' lives (Houston & Diller, 1987) is important. An ethics of care compels Maureen to examine the dynamics of the situation. Maureen, as one caring, does not seek to sit in judgment of Rebecca but rather seeks to enter Rebecca's world in order to see things as Rebecca sees them. When Maureen focused on establishing accountability, by judging, Hoagland (1987) points out, she was involved in a one-way process of examining Rebecca through her, Maureen's, own framework.

Conversely, with what Hoagland (1987) refers to as the two-way process of intelligibility, there is a "presumption of cooperation, not a presumption of antagonism" (p. 36). The concept of intelligibility stems from the work of Marilyn Frye. It ". . . means being willing to situate ourselves in such a way that others who make choices different from ours can be intelligible to us" (p. 35). When Rebecca engages in a dialogue with Maureen, Rebecca becomes involved in the process of self-understanding by beginning to offer explanations (rather than justification) for her choices. Noddings (1984) notes that this kind of dialogue is central to nurturing the ethical ideal. Maureen, as one caring, receives Rebecca. Rebecca, now as one cared for and engaged with her teacher, is able to share and reflect on her own "abilities, defenses, intentions, goals, and needs" (Hoagland, 1986, p. 33). Thus, the process of intelligibility involves both individuals sharing their unique explanations and coming to understand the dynamics of the situation.

Maureen provides Rebecca with learning opportunities that will allow her to engage in a caring encounter with her patient. One means to achieve this end is to share with students the personal accounts of patients, not just the textbook version of what to do when. One example of this can be found in an article by Kelpin (1984) entitled "Birthing Pain." Just as Noddings (1984) cautions us, as one's caring, to "promote skepticism and noninstitutional affiliation" (p. 103), Kelpin urges nurses to heed the voices of women experiencing childbirth pain and to thus be skeptical of their own assumptions about the patients' experiences.

Maureen, in modelling the receptivity of caring, demonstrates to Rebecca the caring relationship between patient and nurse. Maureen helps Rebecca refocus on the experience of the young woman who is about to deliver her baby. Maureen taps into Rebecca's natural tendency to care, which she evidenced in her initial shock at what she had witnessed. Rebecca, according to feminist philosophers Houston and Diller (1987), must be given the opportunity to examine those conditions under which she can trust herself to care. Rebecca is encouraged to continue in her quest for self-knowledge. "The test question then becomes: Can I make known to myself what it is I rely on in trusting my own judgment?" (p. 57).

In the final analysis, it is important to note that an ethics of care does not equate with moral relativism. Right and wrong, Noddings (1984) suggests, can be useful. And there are some things that are clearly wrong. What I am suggesting is that an ethics of care has greater potential for "heightening moral perception and sensitivity in the student" (p. 90). Nurse educators must move away from their tendency to be both judge and jury to their students. They must seek to create a caring dialogue with students that will foster students' ability to make moral choices under conditions of oppression, choices that enhance rather than diminish their vision of themselves as caring practitioners.

REFERENCES

American Nurses' Association. (1985). *Code for nurses with interpretive statements*. Kansas City: ANA

Aristotle. (1976). *Nicomanchean ethics*, Book III. (M. Ostwald, trans.). New York: Norton.

Beauchamp, T. L., & Childress, J. F. (1983). *Principles of biomedical ethics* (2nd ed.). New York: Oxford University Press.

Hersh, R. H., Paolitto, D. P., & Reimer, J. (1979). *Promoting moral growth: From Piaget to Kohlberg.* New York: Longman Inc.

Hoagland, S. L. (1986). Moral agency under oppression. *Trivia, 9,* 73–91.

Hoagland, S. L. (1987). Moral agency under oppression: Beyond praise and blame. *Trivia, 10,* 24–40.

Houston, B., & Diller, A. (1987). Trusting ourselves to care. *Resources for Feminist Research, 16*(3), 35–38.

Kalisch, P. A., & Kalisch, B. J. (1986). *The advance of American nursing.* Boston: Little, Brown.

Kelpin, V. (1984). Birthing pain. *Phenomenology and Pedagogy, 2*(2), 179–187.

Noddings, N. (1984). *Caring: A feminine approach to ethics and moral education.* Berkeley: University of California Press.

Pence, T. (1987). Approaches to nursing ethics. *Philosophy in Context: An Examination of Applied Philosophy, 17,* 7–16.

Pitts, T. (1985). The covert curriculum. *Nursing Outlook, 33*(1), 37–39, 42.

Rich, A. (1976). *Of woman born: Motherhood as experience and institution.* New York: Norton.

Roberts, S. J. (1983). Oppressed group behavior: Implications for nursing. *Advances in Nursing Science, 5*(4), 21–31.

Thompson, J. L. (1987). Critical scholarship: The critique of domination in nursing. *Advances in Nursing Science, 10*(1), 27–39.

Veatch, R. M., & Fry, S. T. (1987). *Case studies in nursing ethics.* London: J. B. Lippincott Company.

Yarling, R. R., & McElmurray, B. J. (1986). The moral foundation of nursing. *Advances in Nursing Science, 8*(2), 63–75.

Reprinted from *Advances in Nursing*, Vol. 11, No 3, pp. 53–61, with permission of Aspen Publishers, Inc., © 1989.

17

Nurse Caring as Constructed Knowledge

Virginia Knowlden

Although several theorists have described care, among them Erickson (1968), Heidegger (1962), and Perry (1970), until Gilligan's (1982) research was published, care and caring as a human virtue was not seen as established until adulthood. Gilligan demonstrated that care and caring in women's development is an important force that shapes women's behavior as early as preadolescence (p. 30). Because previous work in human development had been done almost exclusively on men, Gilligan's work is an important landmark in our knowledge about women, about ourselves as humans.

Belenky et al. (1986) examined women's ways of knowing, and described five different perspectives from which women view reality. These five perspectives—silence, received knowledge, subjective knowledge, procedural knowledge, and constructed knowledge—also represent an evolutionary development of mind and self. The authors drew their perspectives from interviews with ordinary women living ordinary lives. From that examination the authors were able to formulate conclusions about truth, knowledge, authority (p. 3), and expertise (p. 137).

Nurse-practiced caring is knowledge construed from personal experiences in nurse education and practice. In this paper, the data concerning clinical practice is derived from two studies (Knowlden, 1985, 1988) using grounded theory methods as defined by Glaser and Strauss (1967). Data concerning nurse education is drawn from personal experience in nursing practice and education.

Knowlden (1985) defines nurse caring as a form of interpersonal communication between nurses and patients. The complexities of content and interpersonal relationship revealed by the communication are integrated in the nurses' actions. In this study, the content aspects of caring found to be congruent among the nurse and patient participants were health teaching, health assessment, and physical care; the congruent aspects of relationship were showing concern, extending progress and hope, listening, the personal relationship between nurse and patient, building self-esteem, touching, and laughter and humor. According to this framework, caring in nursing does not exist without content and relationship. For example, nursing knowledge directs the nurse's provision of physical care, but without the relationship aspect of feeling concern, or being gentle and careful, or extending a sense of progress and hope, caring is not present in the therapeutic interpersonal nurse–patient relationship. As Knowlden describes it, the patient may be treated, but the person is not cared for.

During the education of the nurse, curriculum content includes aspects of relating in the communication of caring, as they are able to be taught. Once in practice, the content of the nursing education program embedded in the nurse provides a ground for caring actions in the interpersonal relationship between nurse and patient. The embedded nursing knowledge enables the nurse to provide individualized care to a patient.

Belenky et al. (1986) defined constructed knowledge as "a position in which women view all knowledge as contextual, experience themselves as creators of knowledge, and value both subjective and objective strategies for knowing" (p. 15). Knowlden (1988) provides an appropriate example of constructed knowledge drawn from a nurse's response to the videotaped record of her caring for a patient in an ICU.

> Because the patient had a trach, I had to observe her nonverbal behavior to figure out what was going on with her. I knew the minute I walked in the door what kind of day she was having by the expression on her face, and she knew me well, too. I'm explaining things to her; for her that would mean a lot; . . . I'm translating, helping her communicate with other health care workers. I touch her arm. I'm getting closer physically and taking time to understand her. I'm reiterating for clearer communication . . . not being in a rush to go anywhere . . . You don't even have to say anything anymore; you can just read her, empathizing with what she's going through . . . I'm giving her time . . . creating an atmosphere in which she could ask questions and not feel like she was imposing.

The nurse observes and participates in the nursing situation and understands from the context the way in which nursing care is to be delivered. She uses both objectives and subjective strategies for knowing in order to understand the situation and to proceed within its context.

Belenky et al.'s (1986) research revealed that it was introspection about the self in the search for an authentic voice that brought women to the insight that "all knowledge is constructed, and the knower is an intimate part of the known" (p. 137). Constructivist thinkers understand that the answers to questions change with the context in which they are asked, and with the frame of reference of the asker. As a result, there is a "transformation in the understanding of the self which begins to generalize and affect how women think about the truth, knowledge, and expertise. [They] become aware that questions and answers vary through history, across cultures, from discipline to discipline, and from individual to individual" (p. 137). An interview with a nurse from a pediatric intensive care unit, also conducted by Knowlden (1988), disclosed that:

> For the most part, you overlook the tubes as you're so used to them. You deal with the baby as a baby, yet knowing the possibility he'll get into trouble. You get to know the kids by taking care of them for long periods of time . . . It's concentrated care . . . You get to know what the family is feeling about the hospitalization. You care for both, parents and children. You consider what they're dealing with—the babies being in here for so long . . . You talk to the parents; this dad feels so helpless. You explain things as simply as possible as they're so anxious. You [get to] know of the other kids, find out how they [the parents] manage the other children as well who are at home. You make accommodations for the quadruplet at home to visit.

In this situation, the nurse recognizes that the questions and the answers vary from situation to situation, and from individual to individual. Her understanding of her self affects how she thinks about knowledge and experience.

The ability "to see that all knowledge is a construction and that truth is a matter of the context in which it is embedded is to greatly expand the possibilities of how to think about anything, even those things we consider to be the most elementary and obvious" (Belenky et al., 1986, p. 138.) For this nurse, "theories become not truth but models for experience" (p. 138).

Understanding the general tenuousness of knowledge, the importance of their own frame of reference, and their power and ability to construct and reconstruct frames of reference, the women in Belenky et al.'s (1986) study felt "responsible for examining, questioning, and developing the systems that they will use for constructing knowledge. Question posing and problem posing become prominent methods of inquiry, strategies that some researchers have identified as a fifth stage of logical thought" (p. 139). Question posing, central to constructivist knowing, is also at the heart of Gilligan's (1982) responsibility orientation to morality. According to Belenky et al.,

> *Women resolve conflicts through trying to understand the conflict in the context of each person's perspective, needs, and goals —and doing the best possible for everyone (involved) . . . For the constructivist, the moral response is a caring response. The constructivists conviction that they must care and develop "an affinity for the world and the people in it" drives the formation of commitments and eventual action.* (p. 150)

Question posing is revealed in this interview, as reported by Knowlden (1988), with a nurse working in an adult ICU:

> *Caring. It means being concerned, true concern about others' feelings, problems, situations, overall well-being . . . it takes a long time to learn to care; it's not perfected. Sometimes I find myself beyond the point of caring. There's a point to how much you care . . . finally totally emotionally and physically exhausted from trying to give the support, . . . I sit back and say, this could be my family. Would I want this for them?*

She continues, answering a question concerning caring upon admission to the ICU:

> *It is caring, but not in the sense I used before; this caring is doing your job. You can't take time out to truly care, for example, when you're wheeling the patient with a massive MI up from the ER. You care, you have to care to be a nurse, there's some type of caring for every human, but at that point you can't say you truly care; you truly care once you can relate with him. It's your job but if you're not caring, you're not a nurse; you're a burnt-out nurse looking over the tubes to the person. When you're caring, you're there . . . That's caring, verbalizing, eye contact, looking them straight in the eye . . . Now, like with the balloon pump, we're not used to it; one of us said, "I'll take care of the balloon pump, if you'll take care of the patient." Now the main object of my caring is the machine which is taking care of, keeping the patient's life going. You take care of the machine as you don't want to jeopardize that life; it's caring in that way.*

In this example, the nurse is sorting her way through caring, coming to terms with caring and not-caring, as well as professional and technical caring. You can hear her working through her conflict. Her commitment to caring forms the perspective for her eventual actions. Her actions reveal the responsible morality she attempts to practice.

According to Belenky et al. (1986), the majority of the women who use constructivist knowing

> *actively reflect on how their judgments, attitudes, and behavior coalesce into some internal experience of moral consistency . . . they are seriously preoccupied with the moral or spiritual dimension of their lives . . . they strive to translate their moral commitments into action, both out of a conviction that "one must act" and . . . a feeling of responsibility to the larger community . . . (p. 150)*

The above aspects of active reflection, preoccupation with the moral dimension with an impetus toward action, and a feeling of responsibility to the larger community are exemplified by a young nurse in the neonatal ICU as reported by Knowlden (1988):

> My first primary patient had chest tubes, IVs, central lines. We had to do chest compressions. I focused on the parents and their needs; this was taking care of the whole family. They were Jehovah Witnesses and I had to be very, very sensitive in talking to them, especially to the father. I used his feelings to care for the baby as having similar feelings as the father. I was sensitive about the invasive procedures as I became the advocate for the baby as their rights were taken away . . . The parents are your major source to bring you down to the baby, not just taking care of tubes. The parents would just as soon the baby died, but the medical staff didn't feel that way. When giving the baby blood, (the case) had to go to court; medicine could not let the baby die; they had to treat. I have a very different position. I let the parents know that I was in a neutral position. I would be an advocate against aggressive treatment. I would respect their rights. This baby was just transferred to the normal nursery.

In this example, there is also present the struggle to find the "balance between inner and outer authority, . . . the balance between interests" (Belenky et al., 1986, p. 132–33). Once that balance is achieved through her own construction of knowledge of the situation, the nurse's role viś-a-v̀is the parents and medical staff is clear. The example demonstrates as well how in everyday nursing situations nurses face and struggle with serious ethical dilemmas.

Belenky et al. (1986) found that

> *constructivist women aspire to work that contributes to the empower-*
> *ment and improvement in the quality of life of others. More than any*
> *other group of women in their study, constructivists feel a part of the*
> *effort to address with others the burning issues of the day and to*
> *contribute as best they can. They speak of integrating feeling and*
> *care into their work.* (p. 152)

A nurse in a pediatric ICU provides an example of these aspects of constructivist knowing as described by Knowlden (1988):

> *There's really no one way of approaching each family. There's the*
> *same approach to suctioning and IVs, but every family is different.*
> *I'm still learning emotional caring and support through knowing the*
> *family, and being with them all the way through. I try to balance the*
> *discomforts against the parents' anxiety and the services involved. I*
> *try to determine when the child needs more and when he's had*
> *enough. It takes about a day to get control of the mechanical stuff. To*
> *get a feeling of balance, that things will work out; the concern with*
> *the family's comfort takes longer. You control it; you create the bal-*
> *ance to talk more openly about things, to get prepared for the in-*
> *evitable. If you're comfortable, you allay the parents' anxiety. You*
> *take each patient as an individual.*

The nurse's struggles for a balance between conflicting interests is sorted through and works to contribute "to the empowerment and improvement in the quality of life of others" (Belenky et al., 1986).

From these stories of nurses talking about caring, it is clear that the nurses used constructed knowledge to make sense out of what was happening in their practice. As one nurse in the study indicated, it was her observation in a labor and delivery unit as a nursing student that gave her her initial understanding about what it means to care for the technology rather than the patient, and to recoil from those nursing actions.

In baccalaureate programs in nursing in particular, students have a broader formal education in the liberal arts and sciences from which to derive knowledge about the world which can later contribute to developing the constructivist perspective. From my experiences in teaching both undergraduate and graduate nursing students, postclinical conferences when used not as an extension of classroom lecture time, but as time to investigate with the students the meaning of their clinical learning experiences, provide the opportune time for the professor to assist students to move in an evolutionary fashion from silence to constructed knowledge.

Classroom teaching methods which require more individual participation than the lecture method will also enable students to question premises. These interactions between student and teacher assist in "voicing and exploring hitherto unexpressed perspectives of women and others (and are) collaborative, cooperative and interactive" (Culley et al., 1985, p. 15). That form of pedagogy will involve

> students in constructing and evaluating their own education
> . . . and assumes each student has legitimate rights and potential
> contributions to the subject matter. Its goal is to enable students to
> draw on personal and intellectual experiences to build a satisfying
> version of the subject to be used productively in their own lives. [Such]
> techniques involve students in assessment, production, and absorp-
> tion of the material . . . The teacher is the major contributor, the
> creator of structure and delineator of issues, not the sole authority.
> (pp. 30–31)

Nursing education has historically used small group experiences as part of its pedagogy. Meaningful small group discussions, understanding communication and group processes, and the presence of cooperation and collaboration lead students to

> explore and discover personal meanings . . . through interaction
> with other people . . . A learning group discussion is far more ten-
> tative, even halting, in its progress, for it deals not with certainty but
> with search . . . Group discussion does not seek to convince . . .
> [it] seeks to help each . . . to find meaning not existing before.
> (Nelson, 1988)

All of the phases in Peplau's (1970) model of the concept and process of learning come into play in a group's discussion. Carefully formulated, the discussion group can foster students' and teachers' critical thinking ability and continued growth toward the constructivist perspective. Understanding how we integrate our nursing knowledge in our practice enables us to countermand factors such as the "increasing emphasis on technicologic care, the maintenance of an authoritarian framework for provision of health and illness care, and economic competition with the associated imperatives for cost-effective, quantitative (bottom-line) approaches" (Disparti, 1988, p. 18) that threaten caring in nursing.

REFERENCES

Belenky, M. F., Clinchy, B., Goldberger, N., & Tarule, J. (1986). *Women's ways of knowing.* New York: Basic Books.

Culley, Margo, Diamond, A., Edwards, L., Lennox, S., & Portuges, C. (1985). The politics of nurturance. In Culley, Margo, & Portuges, C. (Eds.), *Gendered subjects.* Boston: Routledge & Kegan Paul.

Disparti, J. (1988). Caring and self-care. In G. Caliandro & B. Judkins, (Eds.), *Primary nursing practice.* Boston: Scott, Foresman Co.

Erickson, E. H. (1968). *Identity, youth, & crises.* New York: Norton.

Freire, P. (1981). *Pedagogy of the oppressed.* New York: Continuum Publishing Corporation.

Gilligan, C. (1982). *In a different voice.* Cambridge: Harvard University Press.

Glaser, B., & Strauss, A. (1967). *The discovery of grounded theory: Strategies for qualitative research.* Chicago: Aldine Publishing Co.

Heidegger, M. (1962). *Being and time.* New York: Harper & Row.

Knowlden, V. (1985). *The meaning of caring in the nursing role.* (University Microfilms, Inc. #8525485). *Dissertation Abstracts International,* Vol. 46/09-A, p. 2574.

Knowlden, V. (1988). [Caring in nursing: Is it surviving in high-tech health care settings?] Unpublished research data.

Nelson, C. (1988). *Teaching critical thinking across the disciplines.* Unpublished mimeographed paper. West Hartford, CT: University of Hartford.

Peplau, H. (1970). *Process and concept of learning.* In S. F. Burd & M. A. Marshall (Eds.), *Some clinical approaches to psychiatric nursing.* London: Macmillan.

Perry, W. (1970). *Forms of intellectual and ethical development in the college years.* New York: Holt, Rinehart and Winston.

Seidel, J. V., Kjolseth, R., & Seymour, E. (1988). *The ethnograph (Version 3.0).* Littleton, CO: Qualis Research Associates.

18

A Feminist Analysis of Constructs of Health

Sheila K. Smith

Models of health are essential to nursing. Clarity regarding such models—how our relationships with the larger world will be characterized and where our interests lie—must be attained as well. But this concern is various and expressed through ideological, practical, and, ultimately, personal modes. As a result, constructions of nursing realities hinge on alternative models of health.[1] And to the extent that nursing's constructions reflect and create social realities, nursing's work in this domain has consequences that extend further: to the practices and discourses of society itself.

With regard to health, the nature of desired outcomes, and means for achieving such outcomes, changes in client and care provider roles occur in direct relation to the way health is theorized. For women in patriarchy, where feminist analyses have shown that perpetuation of dominant culture understandings and practices very often results in perpetuation of abuses toward women, this has had significant implications. In effect, there has been gender blindness in regard to nursing's understandings of health, the particular danger of which can be appreciated when juxtaposed with the undermining but often unrecognized gender biases inherent in dominant culture constructions.[2]

Nursing's inquiries into the nature of health have identified the emergence of at least three conceptualizations: health as absence of disease, health as high level wellness, and health as patterning and development.[3] Discussion of these three frameworks has included differentiation on the basis of the understanding of the person and his (sic)[4] relationship to the environment: whether that relationship is characterized as unitary evolvement and mutual simultaneous interaction (Rogers, Parse, Newman, etc.), or whether mechanistic and exchange-type relationships are implied.[5] Sarter (1988) has suggested that it is the former which is emerging as central to nursing's thought patterns. Less attention has been focused on to the functional consequences of various conceptualizations, however; that is, to whose interests are being advanced, whose are being obscured. An explicit connection to feminist theory and perspectives has not been made as well. While the "mutual simultaneous interaction" perspective might suggest the possibility of understanding knowledge development—including knowledge development about health—as an interest-motivated social construction, those who position themselves within this orientation seem not to adopt a social constructionist stance, and may be repeating essentializing moves.[6] The result is that understandings of how health acts as a social construction and representational system get lost in arguments about what constitutes "correct" knowledge of health as a "thing." When health is defined in one specific way and then the claim made that the definition is universalizable, it becomes difficult to explain why the established definition doesn't work in some people's lives. Real differences in people's lives are obscured, as are the ways our theoretical constructions operate in those lives. The understanding that, perhaps, differing and even conflicting definitions of health might be useful for different people at different times and in different situations, becomes hard to sustain. In particular, it becomes difficult to reveal the understanding that health might work with gender in certain ways to structure social life and sustain women's oppression but that, in another sense, women can rework those definitions and practices in politically useful, resistive, and subversive ways.[7]

In this paper I will examine alternative constructions of "health" and the epistemology that informs them. Based on this analysis, I hope to reach conclusions regarding the adequacy of the various constructs from a feminist perspective. I will describe the three perspectives on health mentioned previously and compare them from their respective ontological/epistemological perspectives. In addition, I will discuss them from a feminist perspective in terms of consequences for the individual and nursing. Finally, I will present considerations in thinking about women's health from a feminist perspective on the authoritative self as interconnected, in-relation, and idiosyncratic.

NURSING, HEALTH, AND GENDER

The natural world is inexorably routine. Bodies wear out and die like flowers, dark follows light, rivers flow down, trees grow up, new birth emerges from decay. There is no controlling this process. It just goes on and on. The human animal comes into this world in a certain time and place. We are neither the center, nor the beginning, nor the end. We are only one manifestation of life. (Cheatham & Powell, 1986, p. 159)

The attitude conveyed by Cheatham and Powell is a reality known well to nurses: the coming and going of human lives; the fragile rhythms of birthing, growing, failing, and dying; connecting and separating. This would seem to be the natural-world process of health: the movement and diversity of trans-forming patterns of energy exchange; the complexity and idiosyncrasy of the processes of human lives. Nurses know this world intimately. We mediate the transitions, reveal the possibilities, mobilize the resources, negotiate the passages, guide the choices. Nursing becomes the work of connecting-interpreting, facilitating sense-making, and meaningful world-negotiating approaches in regard to the ways we live in this world through our bodies.[8]

However, I believe that nurses idealize when nursing theories attend to this process from an individualistic and naturalized perspective, ignoring the acted-out social processes within which people's health and nursing occurs. Sometimes we do a magnificent job, facilitating the other's transformations in patterning through our own direct engagement in the trajectory of their life processes. At other times, however, we fail miserably, reducing others to objects, denying the possibility of their subjectivity, excluding their own experiencing of their health patterning. There is a distinct difference in the quality of interactions in these two scenarios. The difference can be attributed partially to one's understanding of health: whether one accepts the dominant cultural perspective, arising out of Cartesian separation of self and world, or an alternative perspective, based on an understanding of persons as embodied and connected. But explaining the difference seems to require an understanding of the social processes at work as well. The first scenario—the engagement scenario, and nursing's preferred scenario—seems more common in regard to women's health when a politicized, connected perspective is embraced. I don't believe we've been very clear about this difference, and we certainly haven't done much in terms of understanding its implications from the standpoint of those of us who are embodied as female. The paradigm of health emerging out of nursing concerns the lived experience of health for specific persons in specific situations. What this paradigm has not taken notice of, however, is that when the specific persons are women, the lived experience is one regulated by the workings of gender.

Focusing on the workings of gender in social processes is the specific domain of feminist theory. Feminist theory examines misshapen and oppressive gender arrangements and the distortions they create in women's lives, trying "to make the experiences and lives of women intelligible" (Frye, 1983, p. xi). Thompson (1987) has described critical theory as a process of thinking and acting in a manner that challenges institutionalized power relations and relations of domination. As a gender-specific form of critical theory, the same can be said of feminism. Like critical theory (again borrowing from Thompson), the implications of feminist theory are important for the social institution and discipline of nursing, as well as for social definitions and practices of health: its promise is the possibility of transforming the social world toward affirmation of women's lived experiences and active participation in the construction of reality. As applied to phenomena of concern to nursing, the promise becomes the possibility of transforming women's lived experiences and meanings of health and health care.

INSTITUTIONALIZED, SOCIALLY DOMINANT
PERSPECTIVES OF HEALTH

The socially dominant model of health is biomedical in form and structure. This model of health has come to include both health as absence of disease and, through expropriation, health as complete well-being.

Several nursing authors have presented critiques of the biomedical model in relation to nursing's declared orientation toward persons and health.[9] Allen (1986) and Lyddon (1987) have described how the operant philosophic orientation in health as absence of disease is functional-analytic, based on an essentialist definition. Within this understanding, and to some extent within our general cultural consciousness, the essence of health has come to be regarded as the absence of disease, wherein disease has attained a separate ontologic status as a reified "thing." The essentialist view of health as absence of disease implies the objective, empirically verifiable existence of health as unitary, separate from the individual person and societal meanings, describable in terms of certain features, and identifiable quite simply in terms of its presence or absence (Allen, 1986). As health in this perspective is dependent on absence of disease, disease is granted ontological priority. Both health (as absence of disease) and disease (as that whose presence denies the existence of health) are studied in a positivist framework of reductionism, unidimensionality, linearity, and cause and effect relationships. Disease becomes viewed as a mutually exclusive taxonomy for which single causes and specific cures can be identified—the application of which extinguishes disease, leaving health.

The definition of health as complete well-being provides only slight variation on this perspective—seemingly, it still falls within the essentialist framework. Health as complete well-being assumes a continuum format, establishing a polarity between disease and high-level wellness (health), with high-level wellness occupying the position held by absence of disease in the former model. Adaptation to disease and absence of disease apparently lie somewhere between the two extremes (Newman, 1986; Smith, 1981). Newman (1986) has specifically objected to the adequacy of this model for nursing. Several others (Bramwell, 1984; Peplau, 1988; Watson, 1988) have implied an agreement with Newman's position.

Although the essentialist nature of health as complete well-being is less evident than in health as absence of disease, I would argue that it is present nonetheless, and perhaps in a more insidious form. The difference concerns one element: the exclusionary perspective has been expanded, and considerably so. Now, health is not just absence of disease, but the absence of all factors that would threaten complete well-being: physical, psychological, social, spiritual, relational, environmental, economic, and so on. The "normal," highly sought, and institutionally correct state of health is not only free of disease, but normatively imbued with white, middle class, male privilege.

Without careful, critical analysis, the perspective of health as complete well-being seems quite appealing. It also seems to create the possibility of an understanding of health that extends beyond the physiologic realm to include domains of person and environment. Seemingly, it might allow more persons to believe themselves "healthy," as a broader, more complexly integrated domain of characteristics is included in the definition. It appeals to our understanding that health is not just about the physical body, but about the person and his or her lived world: functional capacity, coping strategies, social support network, access to resources, self-actualization, and quality of life. Schlotfeldt (1987a, 1987b) and Smith (1981) identify this perspective as dominant in nursing: it seems to represent health as a relative and holistic construct, recognizing the person-to-person variability in states of health.

My own sense, however, is that the continuum model is illusory. It does not represent a liberating perspective of health. Rather, the view of health it depicts is unavailable to all but the most privileged, and perhaps, most conforming.[10] The regions between disease (as that which marks incapacitation and loss of independence) and complete well-being may reflect some degree of health, but more trenchantly reflect escalating emphasis on disease, limitation, and deviance as that which defines the individual. As Sontag (1978) explains, the problem is that these liminal regions are not identified as socially accept-able places to inhabit. The ultimate, standardized goal remains health, which as complete well-being becomes virtually unattainable. Disease retains its same negative polarity (Newman, 1986), assigning the person-bearers of that label to the same socially marginalized, devalued place as in the perspective of health as absence of disease. In the name of liberalism, however, those who reside in the borderlands between complete well-being and incapacitating disease are al-lowed to "pass" as healthy, as long as they can successfully disguise the embar-rassing fact of their illness, or atone for it by superhuman performance in other socially ratified realms (Register, 1987).[11]

EPISTEMOLOGIC BASIS FOR THE BIOMEDICAL
MODELS OF HEALTH

How did these biased, oppressive ideas of health achieve their socially ac-cepted status? Feminist theorists (Bordo, 1986; Grimshaw, 1986, 1988; Lloyd, 1984; Ruth, 1981; Scheman, 1983, in press; Young-Bruehl, 1987) suggest that an appropriate place to begin such analyses is from an historical and philo-sophical perspective: from culturally transmitted thought forms and habits of construction, "obstacles that have deep roots—in our culture and in our-selves" (Young-Bruehl, 1987, p. 220).

Descartes' project has been identified as crucial to these habits (Bordo, 1986; Grimshaw, 1988; Hodge, 1988; Lloyd, 1984).[12] Although thoroughly entangled in an historical context of reflexive social consciousness, Descartes' philosophy identified what was problematic for much of modern Western philosophy (Flax, 1983; Griffiths, 1988; Hodge, 1988; Scheman, 1983): what it is that distinguishes the knowing subject, and the process for attaining this distinction. His solution to these problems had a considerable influence on establishing in Western culture the hierarchical relationship of rationality over experience, the separation and stratification of mind and body, and the essen-tial distinctness of persons. Within this framework, that which is associated with female is located in the immanent, the concrete, the particular (as op-posed to the transcendent, the abstract, the universal)—that which needs to be strictly controlled, and so that which is justifiably subordinated, devalued (Griffiths, 1988).

The Cartesian method is based on the belief that there is an objectively correct knowledge about the world, accessible to the unencumbered self. What prevents the mind from knowing the world correctly, from being an authorita-tive self in understanding the world, is embodiment in the concrete, experien-tial world. To overcome this obstacle, Descartes proposed methical doubt about all things as "a very simple way by which the mind may detach itself from the senses" (Descartes, 1968, p. 140). Radically separating the mind from the body, withdrawing from the world, isolating the self from external, physical distraction, is postulated to result in objective clarity. When detached from the world, the self can achieve understanding of basic, universal truths. True knowledge of the world is based on dispassionate detachment and clear separation of self from not-self.[13]

The consequences of the Cartesian method have been politically and epistemically oppressive (Hodge, 1988; Scheman, 1983, in press). Control and separation resulted in views of selves as fundamentally isolated, disconnected; in devaluing, doubting the experiential world of embodiment, relationship, sense experience, and diversity; and in granting epistemic authority to those who are not different, those who can claim knowledge of the unitary realm, those who reside in transcendent sameness, while denying it to all others. That which is denied as unknowable, relegated to the not-self, is also that which has been attributed to the female way of being in the world: that which is experiential, idiosyncratic, reciprocal, intimate, interdependent, and vulnerable. Significantly, the privilege of epistemic authority was not extended to women.[14]

In the ontologic perspective where one kind of truth predominates, political hegemony is also legitimated, extending the normative privilege of hierarchical authority to all human constructions of reality (Scheman, in press; Young-Bruehl, 1987). The political effect of this difference-denying stance on individuals is revealed in systematic patterns of denial, victimization, and marginalization. I would contend that these patterns are revealed in understandings of health, and are particularly revealing when considering the possibility of health for women.

RELATIONSHIP TO MODELS OF HEALTH

Representations of health in the biomedical model are fully embedded in mind–body duality and transcendent beliefs about authoritative, empowered selves. As part of a complex political process, granted legitimacy in part through the modernist orientation toward analytical, reductionistic thinking as the most advanced and valuable form, health has come to be equated with medicalism. Other approaches are derided and institutionally invalidated as nonrational and nonscientific.[15]

It is relevant here to consider the word *heal*, the supposed process of health, meaning *to make whole* (Keller, 1981). Under medicalism, this is equated with the undisturbed functioning of the mechanistic body. The Cartesian self, that separates from objectifies, and controls its own body, still finds this body indispensable (Scheman, in press). Succumbing to disease, or even disturbing the mechanistic body through a process that is not disease, is regarded as failure of the body, indicating failure of control, failure of the self. If the failure is one that can be repaired, the self can be salvaged, except—as Scheman (in press) notes—for the embarrassment of having sustained an injury and the weakness or flaw of self it might imply. But, in general, no substantial deviation of the sameness of this self from the normative, authoritative self is announced. This has been the epistemic role of the biomedical approach: to sustain the undisturbed functioning of the mechanistic body, or at least to sustain the appearance of undisturbed functioning, in order that the self may claim wholeness and sameness.

If the failure cannot be repaired, epistemic authority is quickly lost. The difference between this self and the normative, unflawed self cannot be denied. It becomes a nearly impossible task to separate self from a body that won't disappear, so to speak: that demands constant attention to maintain some semblance of "normal" functioning, that won't abide by the socially defined rules of control, or that persists in messy, uncomfortable, unresponsive, and unsolicited sensory activities. This body—marked by transgressions of sensation, inconstancy, and constraint—is a bit too close to immanence and unreliability, and is alien to an unencumbered self. To be ill or disabled—to lack health—is often to be disempowered and perceived as lacking in competence (Zegans, 1987).

As the biomedical system is a politically empowered system, the loss of epistemic authority carries with it the loss of unquestioned, privileged access to many of society's places of power, including, ironically, to health care. The chronically ill, the elderly, the disabled, and impoverished women with children unsponsored by men become part of the marginalized many whose access to health care is far from ensured.

Defining health as complete well-being does not improve things. This model, in fact, seems to approach the paranoid extreme of Cartesian dualism: marginalization can be justified on the failure of self to attain problem-free, decontextualized existence in multiple domains.[16] The transcendent project shifts from transcending embodiment to transcending all that is disagreeable or complicated about our lived experiences—an option clearly not available to most women in this world.

Similarities can be noted when this thinking about the transgressive, unreliably embodied, encumbered self and possibilities for health is extended to thinking about women and health. To the extent that the disadvantaging of and disregard for the unhealthy body is related to its immanence, its insistence on the experiential, and that the same weakness is also attributed to what seems to be embodied as female, women's attempts to claim health become appropriated by culture. Established cultural constructs of body, self, and health are not, for women, a mutually sustaining and complementary trio working toward the realization of human excellence. Rather, body, self, and health become fragmented: the contradictory and incongruous site of female sexualization (Haug, 1987). Desire and objectification become confused, making health less clearly intelligible.

NURSING'S ALTERNATIVE CONSTRUCTS OF HEALTH

The domain of concern in nursing is the embodied self precisely—the lived experiences of immersion in the world and connectedness to others through a locus of idiosyncrasies that is, among other aspects, physical. Because this is not an orientation given much regard under Cartesian dominance, the consequences for nursing are clearly visible in its positioning in the health care system. Nursing's socially defined primary role has been to support and complement medical care—never mind that this role places nurses daily in morally indefensible positions in relation to clients. However, the understanding of health emerging in nursing is qualitative, idiosyncratic, and contextual. It is concerned with illness as one manifestation of the patterning in people's lives; as a significant part of their experience of wholeness, rather than as a detriment to wholeness (Newman, 1986). What nursing has failed to include is an understanding that those experiences are also gendered.

Our experience of living is embodied experience. Our participation in the world and connectedness to others is only possible through our physical construction. Epistemic authority is not possible apart from our existence in the world as physical beings. With this understanding, the lived experience of health, in whatever diverse and changing manner it may be manifested, is worth paying attention to, worth making accessible to the individual as their idiosyncratic way of being immersed in the world. Intentional engagement in the embodied, rhythmical transformations of health can attribute legitimate subjectivity to persons who've previously had that privilege denied. In recently developed nursing theory, health is not just the absence of disease, or the achievement of biopsychosocial well-being, but the lived manifestations of one's constitution in the world (Newman, 1986; Parse, 1981). Feminist analyses make clear, however, that women's embodiment is

not a coequal matter: women's rights to individual bodily integrity—as
part of that assigned to the private realm—are often not under women's
control.[17]

CRITIQUE IN FEMINIST TERMS

In an unsettling way, the works of the above nurse theorists seem to be
characterized by equalizing and essentializing tendencies similar to those in
the model health as absence of disease. Rather than appealing to a mechanized
model of man (sic), they appeal to ecologic models of a unitary unfolding.
Women's lives, however, marked by the workings of gender, seem sometimes
to be more about experiences of fragmentation, discrepancy, and alienation
than about transcendence and evolvution.

The understanding of health as lived experience is potentially a feminist,
liberating perspective. It supports inclusiveness and celebration of differences.
It constructs the self as interconnected, in-relation, and idiosyncratic. It engages inquiry in processes of attention to contextual detail, patterns of interconnection, and particularity. And it creates the possibility of a radical
coalition politic among those whose epistemic authority and privileged access
to health care was previously denied, by recognizing the legitimacy of their full
participation in the construction of reality. Proclaiming that legitimacy and
describing what is, in fact, the situation in the world are two different things,
however. Missing from the discussion so far is a gender-based analysis of how
these processes might work specifically for women, including an understanding of the complexity of women's fragmented experiences and oppositional
struggles we sustain in order to understand ourselves as relatively coherent
and whole. A more adequate basis for theory about health for women might
be to recognize how women's processes of health require close attendance and
management of fragments;[18] and, perhaps, that facilitating different understandings of health in different situations might turn out to be very useful for
women. Some women may be well served by cured disease, others by improved functional status, some by pattern explication, still others by physical
protection from harm or the facilitation of access to reproductive control.
Comparing totalizing definitions of health for a single, more adequate understanding becomes a confusion because, as Register (1987) puts it in regard to
disease, ". . . there is no single basis for it—not the severity of pain or
disability, not the number of years of ill health endured, not even the likeli-
hood of death" (p. xiv). Nor, I would add, is there a single basis for it in regard
to the social processes in which women's lives are grounded, the amount

of damage done by problems we know specifically to be foregrounded in discussions of health for women, arising from our embodiment and objectification as female.

Taking refuge in a mind–body split is perhaps equally difficult and, as Register (1987) points out, a delusion, when "healthy" and "normal" are androcentric social constructs equated with perfection. Imperfection and encumbrance are, of course, the more representative rules, but somehow that simple observation has gotten lost in our general cultural consciousness. How do we construct norms to reflect imperfection, diversity, and recovery? How do we go about the social process of reclaiming, revaluing less than perfect and sometimes violated bodies as a legitimate place from which to declare an experience of the world? This seems to be one of the problems taken up by nursing. When the subject of that theory are women, however, I do not believe that models of unitary unfolding are an adequate conceptual place from which to begin. Embodiment as female is perilous business. As with persons who live with illness, women who've experienced first hand the destructiveness of our lack of meaningful control of embodiment face real threats to self. Relationships to specific others and community, work and financial stability, and functional self-maintenance all become shaded, not so much by the uncertainty of biologic processes that resist stability (although this, too, becomes problematic for some), but by the struggle to interpret discrepant experiences of self in the world.

Newman (1986) identifies the process of health as expanding consciousness: increasing the quality and diversity of person–environment interactions. Health is not objectified as physiologic process or absence of disease, but as a qualitative reflection of pattern in person–environment interaction. Intentional engagement with the embodied, rhythmical transformations of health can attribute legitimate subjectivity to persons who've previously had this privilege denied.

Nonetheless, I do have significant difficulty with the above conceptualization. Transcendence and connectedness are not clearly differentiated, also I'm suspicious of projects considered transcendent.[19] Newman would also like to set aside the understanding of health as a positive evaluative indicator, accepting the patterning of all persons, in all manner of diverse manifestations, as health for that person. While I think I know what Newman means and have a sense of how to do this when the person's manifestation of health is privatized as personal disease, I have great difficulty understanding how this works with the specifically nonprivate social health problems around control of sexuality, for which it seems there is great political and conceptual use in retaining the evaluative meaning of health.

Parse (1981; and Parse, Coyne, & Smith, 1985) discusses themes of energy, plentitude, harmony. Parse's characterizations seem somehow too idealized and privileged, however: excluding those who don't experience their health as energy and plentitude, privileging the experiences of those who do. Her continued use of the male referent as generic is problematic for me as well. It has been repeatedly well-argued that there is nothing generic about the word *man*, so I am left not knowing to whom, precisely, the work is meant to apply.

Frye (1983) provides some methodologic assistance in developing conceptual schemes that better account for women's experiences. She focuses attention on the basic concepts of self and other not through ontology, as required by the notion of unitary whole, but through a metaphorical and political distinction between the arrogant eye and the loving eye: whether one defines and remakes another with reference to self and one's own interests, resulting—regardless of how unintentional—in a macroeffect of a certain amount of coercion and erasure; or whether one knows boundaries of self and other clearly enough to allow the other their independence, their complexity, and their ability to make their own meaning. For women to make their own meanings in regard to health, however, the workings of gender must be more fully considered.

NOTES

[1] See, for example, Newman's (in press) discussion of interpretive difficulties that arise when conceptual distinctions on health are not mutually clarified.

[2] Important exceptions to this gender blindness can be seen in Campbell (1981, 1986), Duffy (1984), MacPherson (1985), McBride & McBride (1982), Rose (1990), and Woods et al. (1988). Some of these authors, however, characterize gender as not so much about institutionalized power arrangements as about difference. See MacKinnon (1987) for a critique of conceptualizing gender as difference.

[3] Various writers frame this characterization differently. Smith (1981) described four models of health: eudiamonistic, adaptive, role-performance, and clinical. Laffrey, Loveland-Cherry, & Winkler (1986) identified two major paradigms: pathogenic and health; Newman (1986) identified the "old paradigm" as absence of disease, the prevailing view as a health-illness continuum, and the "new paradigm" as a paradigm of pattern. Parse (1987) has identified "totality" and "simultaneity" paradigms.

[4] "His" is used here doubly to draw critical attention to the presumably gender-neutral sense with which nurse writers often refer to persons as

undifferentiated by gender, inclusive of both women and men, as well as to make the claim that such presumptions of gender-neutrality erase the very gendered determination of women's lives.

[5] See Allan & Hall (1988), Connors (1980), Newman (1986, in press), and Sandelowski (1988) for various parts of this analysis.

[6] Allen (1986) discusses the problems of essentializing. I say more about this later, but here I would point out the exclusionary and distorting effect of failing to acknowledge theory and knowledge as social constructions developed to some purpose—a necessary step if one is to sustain any kind of ideological resistance to dominant paradigms. I am referring here both to biomedical models which define health exclusively (or nearly so) as absence of disease and nursing models which define health as processes of unitary unfolding. As a result, health continues to be described as some kind of naturally occurring, i.e. pre-social, ahistorical, monolithic state. This is particularly confusing from a nursing perspective because of our claims to include social dimensions in our understandings of health.

[7] See de Lauretis (1986), Felski (1989), and Harding (1987) on the importance of resistance in feminist thinking.

[8] I link this understanding of nursing to Newman's (in press, 1986) work on patterning and pattern recognition, even though, as I think will become clear, I have difficulty with some other assumptions underlying Newman's thinking.

[9] See note 5.

[10] Wright (1982) discusses how labels of healthy or unhealthy appear to be about organic processes of disease, but in fact operate as markers of conformity to the norms of social organization. Register's (1987) work chronicles how this operates for persons with chronic illness.

[11] Scheman (in press) discusses the problem of liberalism as declaring an essential equality and sameness between persons via the appearance of extending the full notion of rationality and rights, but without really deconstructing the underlying power structures. This is a disempowering move because it acts to placate by obscuring socially and historically constructed hierarchies of control and domination, thereby undermining possibilities for effective resistance.

[12] Flax (1983) traces this establishment of dichotomies and stratification back to Plato. The point remains, however, that the patterns are old and deeply entrenched in our understandings and social structures. Descartes' work seems to mark the point at which these understandings became fixed into modern thinking (Grimshaw, 1988).

[13] This was never postulated as an option available to women, however (Bordo, 1986; Hodge, 1988; Ruth, 1981).

[14] Hughes (1988) traces this exclusion of women from epistemic authority to Aristotle.

[15] This is revealed in licensing laws and practice acts, reimbursement structures, and court cases which punish people for choosing not to seek biomedical health care for their dependents.

[16] Scheman (1983) discusses this as the paranoid extreme of Descartian dualism. See also Bordo (1986), Lloyd (1984), and Ruth (1981).

[17] See Barry (1979), Coward (1985), MacKinnon (1987), Russell and van de Ven (1976).

[18] Thanks go to Ruth Ellen Joeres, M. J. Maynes, and Jacquelyn Zita for helping clarify this in my thinking. See de Lauretis (1986), Felski (1989), Grimshaw (1986, 1988), and Harding (1987).

[19] Newman argues with me about the meaning of her use of the idea of transcendence. She is very clear—and, of course, it makes sense in the context of her writing—that her discussion of transcendence as an element of expanding consciousness is *not* about transcendence in the Cartesian sense. I still have confusion with all of this, however, because of the centrality of the Cartesian sense of the word in my own mind. Through feminist analysis, I have come to regard transcendence as nearly the antithesis of women's everyday lives.

REFERENCES

Allan, J. D., & Hall, B. A. (1988). Challenging the focus on technology: A critique of the medical model in a changing health care system. *Advances in Nursing Science, 10*(3), 22–34.

Allen, D. G. (1986). Using philosophical and historical methodologies to understand the concept of health. In P. L. Chinn (Ed.), *Nursing research methodology: Issues and implementation*. Rockville, MD: Aspen.

Barry, K. (1979). *Female sexual slavery*. Englewood Cliffs, NJ: Prentice-Hall.

Bordo, S. (1986). The Cartesian masculinization of thought. *Signs, 11*, 439–56.

Bramwell, L. (1984). Use of life history in pattern identification and health promotion. *Advances in Nursing Science, 7*(1), 37–44.

Campbell, J. (1981). Misogyny and the homicide of women. *Advances in Nursing Science, 3*(2), 67–85.

Campbell, J. (1986). A survivor group for battered women. *Advances in Nursing Science, 8*(2), 13-20.

Cheatham, A., & Powell, M. C. (1986). *This way daybreak comes: Women's values and the future.* Philadelphia: New Society Publishers.

Connors, D. D. (1980). Sickness unto death: Medicine as mythic, necrophilic, and iatrongenic. *Advances in Nursing Science, 2*(3), 39-51.

Coward, R. (1985). *Female desires.* New York: Grove Press.

de Lauetis, T. (Ed.). (1986). *Feminist studies: Critical studies.* Bloomington: Indiana University Press.

Descartes, R. (1968). *Discourse on method.* Baltimore: Penguin.

Duffy, M. (1984). Transcending options: Creating a milieu for practicing high level wellness. *Health Care for Women International, 5,* 145-161.

Felski, R. (1989). *Beyond feminist aesthetics: Feminist literature and social change.* Cambridge: Harvard University Press.

Flax, J. (1983). Political philosophy and the patriarchal unconscious: A psychoanalytic perspective on epistemology and metaphysics. In S. Harding & M. B. Hintikka (Eds.), *Discovering reality: Feminist perspectives on epistemology, metaphysics, methodology, and philosophy of science.* Dordrecht, Holland: D. Reidel.

Frye, M. (1983). *The politics of reality.* Freedom, CA: Crossing Press.

Griffiths, M. (1988). Feminism, feelings, and philosophy. In M. Griffiths & M. Whitford (Eds.), *Feminist perspectives in philosophy.* Bloomington: Indiana University Press.

Grimshaw, J. (1986). *Philosophy and feminist thinking.* Minneapolis: University of Minnesota Press.

Grimshaw, J. (1988). Autonomy and identity in feminist thinking. In M. Griffiths & M. Whitford (Eds.), *Feminist perspectives in philosophy.* Bloomington: Indiana University Press.

Harding, S. (Ed.). (1987). *Feminism and methodology.* Bloomington: Indiana University Press.

Haug, F. (Ed.). (1987). *Female sexualization: A collective work of memory.* London: Verso.

Hodge, J. (1988). Subject, body and the exclusion of women from philosophy. In M. Griffiths & M. Whitford (Eds.), *Feminist perspectives in philosophy.* Bloomington: Indiana University Press.

Hughes, J. (1988). The philosopher's child. In M. Griffiths & M. Whitford (Eds.), *Feminist perspectives in philosophy.* Bloomington: Indiana University Press.

Keller, M. J. (1981). Toward a definition of health. *Advances in Nursing Science, 4*(1), 43–64.

Laffrey, S. C., Loveland-Cherry, C. J., & Winkler, S. J. (1986). Health behavior: Evolution of two paradigms. *Public Health Nursing, 3*(2), 92–100.

Lloyd, G. (1984). *The man of reason: Male and female in western philosophy.* London: Methuen.

Lyddon, W. J. (1987). Emerging views of health: A challenge to rationalist doctrines of medical thought. *Journal of Mind and Behavior, 8*(3), 365–394.

MacKinnon, C. A. (1987). *Feminism unmodified.* Cambridge: Harvard University Press.

MacPherson, K. I. (1985). Osteoporosis and menopause: A feminist analysis of the social construction of a syndrome. *Advances in Nursing Science, 7*(4), 11–22.

McBride, A. B., & McBride, W. L. (1982). Theoretical underpinnings for women's health. *Women & Health, 6*(1 ½), 37–55.

Newman, M. (in press). Nursing paradigms and realities. In N. Chaska (Ed.), *The nursing profession: Turning points.* New York: McGraw-Hill.

Newman, M. A. (1986). *Health as expanding consciousness.* St. Louis: C. V. Mosby.

Parse, R. R. (1981). *Man-Living-Health: A theory of nursing.* New York: John Wiley & Sons.

Parse, R. R. (1987). *Nursing Science: Major paradigms, theories, and critiques.* Philadelphia: W. B. Saunders.

Parse, R. R., Coyne, A. B., & Smith, M. J. (1985). The lived experience of health: A phenomenologic study. *Nursing research qualitative methods.* MD: Brady Communications.

Peplau, H. E. (1988). The art and science of nursing: Similarities, differences, and relations. *Nursing Science Quarterly, 1*(1), 8–15.

Register, C. (1987). *Living with chronic illness.* New York: Free Press.

Rose, J. F. (1990). Psychologic health for women: A phenomenologic study of women's inner strength. *Advances in Nursing Science, 12*(2), 56–70.

Russell, D. E. H., & van de Ven, N. (1976). *The proceedings of the international tribunal on crimes against women.* Milbrae, CA: Les Femmes.

Ruth, S. (1981). Methodocracy, misogyny, and bad faith: The response of philosophy. In D. Spender (Ed.), *Men's studies modified: The impact of feminism on the academic disciplines.* New York: Pergamon Press.

Sandelowski, M. (1988). A case of conflicting paradigms: Nursing and reproductive technology. *Advances in Nursing Science, 10*(3), 35–45.

Sarter, B. (1988). *The stream of becoming: A study of Martha Rogers' theory.* New York: National League for Nursing.

Scheman, N. (1983). Individualism and the objects of psychology. In S. Harding & M. B. Hintikka (Eds.), *Discovering reality: Feminist perspectives on epistemology, metaphysics, methodology, and philosophy of science.* Dordrecht, Holland: D. Reidel.

Scheman, N. (in press). The body politic/The impolitic body/Bodily politics. In H. U. Gumbrecht & L. Pfeiffer (Eds.), *Materialities of communication.* Cambridge: Harvard University Press.

Schlotfeldt, R. M. (1987a). Defining nursing: A historic controversy. *Nursing Research, 36*(1), 64–67.

Schlotfeldt, R. M. (1987b). Resolution of issues: An imperative for creating nursing's future. *Journal of Professional Nursing, 3,* 136–42.

Sontag, S. (1978). *Illness as metaphor.* New York: Farrar, Straus, & Giroux.

Smith, J. (1981). The idea of health: A philosophic inquiry. *Advances in Nursing Science, 3*(3), 43–50.

Thompson, J. L. (1987). Critical scholarship: The critique of domination in nursing. *Advances in Nursing Science, 10*(1), 27–38.

Watson, J. (1988). New dimensions in human caring theory. *Nursing Science Quarterly, 1*(4), 175–81.

Woods, N. F., Laffrey, S., Duffy, M., Lentz, M. J., Mitchell, E. S., Taylor, D., & Cowan, K. A. (1988). Being healthy: Women's Images. *Advances in Nursing Science, 11*(1), 36–46.

Wright, W. (1982). *The social logic of health.* New Brunswick: Rutgers University Press.

Young-Bruehl, E. (1987). The education of women as philosophers. *Signs, 12,* 207–21.

Zegans, L. S. (1987). The embodied self: Personal integration in health and illness. *Advances, 4,* 29–45.

19

Researching: Designing Research from a Feminist Perspective

Barbara A. Hedin and Mary E. Duffy

This paper focuses on the process of designing a feminist research study. The specific implication that this process differs from that of designing a "traditional research study"—or whatever the counterpart to a feminist study might be—is, to our way of thinking, correct. When operating through feminist consciousness, the author will reflect that consciousness or worldview in the conceptualization and implementation of the research study. But what, in fact, characterizes a feminist engagement with the research process.

Discussions of a feminist research approach or a feminist science evolve out of a feminist critique of positivist science already well-documented in numerous other sources. In the interest of time, I will not detail those arguments here (Bleier, 1986; Fee, 1986; Harding, 1986; Namenwirth, 1986; Stanley & Wise, 1983). However, it is important to recognize that a single feminist critique—"single," that is, in the sense of agreed on by all feminists—does not exist.

Nonetheless, Mary Duffy and I felt a need to reconceptualize the research process in terms sufficiently dynamic to reveal the contradictions and tensions within it (what we mean by this will become clearer as we proceed). While the research process is still presented as a linear sequence in this paper—the limitations of our language—anyone who has conducted research knows that it

227

is only an illusion that one moves lock-step through the process. Initially important, however, to a feminist research process are principles on which it rests.

The design of a feminist research study is informed by several assumptions. Of particular importance is the primary "process assumption" that the means reflect the ends and vice versa. Feminist research is carried out in an emancipatory interest: the aim is enlightenment and more specifically, the empowerment of women and the transformation of patriarchal structures and relations that perpetuate the oppression of women. Therefore, the process itself will reflect both these elements. Equality is at the root of a feminist consciousness as well as horizontally vs. hierarchically structured relations. Feminist research concerns itself with issues that are of vital concern to women or, as Cook and Fonow (1986) state, it sensitizes one to "gender and gender asymmetry as a basic feature of all social life" (p. 5). As such, feminist research starts from the lived experiences of women and does not deny or denigrate the personal, but seeks to validate the private, emotional, and interior world of individuals. Feminist research utilizes a "conscious partiality"—it rejects the subject/object dichotomy and recognizes that personal values play an inherent part in any research endeavor. To maintain clarity, the researcher seeks to make such values explicit to assess their influence on the study, study participants, analysis, and so on, and to take steps to minimize their effects. The researcher also seeks to make such values explicit to the readers/research consumers so that they can evaluate the study for such biases as well. Feminist research also incorporates a recognition of the ethical implications of research and guards against the exploitation of women as objects of research or mere providers of data.

Any particular methodology is not inherently feminist or nonfeminist: it is the intent and means with which it is employed that determines its appropriateness. Cook and Fonow (1986) provide an in-depth discussion of various research methodologies that have been utilized in innovative ways in feminist sociological research studies that can be a fruitful source of ideas for nurse researchers.

RECONCEPTUALIZING THE RESEARCH PROCESS

From having done research, we know the research process is anything but a neat, linear process as discussed in most texts. It is more often experienced as a dynamic, emergent, changing, and tension-filled process. These dynamic qualities are important to recognize and understand. As such we have modelled our work on that of Rowan's (1981), who labels the respective stages of the process we name Researching as: *Being, Thinking, Designing, Encountering, Making Sense,* and *Communicating.*

Following is a description of what each phase entails, then questions that can be asked during each phase to heighten individual awareness of the issues of central importance during each.

The *Being* Phase

Being denotes the phase of researching in which the researcher recognizes that his or her present practice is inadequate and "off the mark" as it were. Dissatisfaction and dissonance with current ways of handling issues, with current practices, also appear. This results in a rejection of current methods of dealing with issues, present ideas, and a sense that things could be different. Feminist research acknowledges the importance of the personal, and is rooted in the lived experiences of women, hence, it pays attention to these dissonant feelings, gives them credence, and uses them as the basis to explore new alternatives.

Questions for Reflection during the Being Phase:[1]

1. Based on an analysis of the situation using all types of knowledge—empirical, personal, aesthetic, and so forth—what do I think is the problem needing analysis, and what do I believe is happening?

2. What contextual factors are affecting the problem?

3. What societal/system factors are affecting this group of women?

4. How do I think the problem could be reconceptualized so that individual women would not be blamed or victimized for not conforming to society?

5. To whom is the problem's solutions relevant?

6. What is my interest in investigating this issue?

7. Does the issue direct attention to issues of sex and gender?

(Duffy & Hedin, 1988, p. 534)

The *Thinking* Phase

The *Thinking* phase is the creative, idea-generating stage in which the researcher seeks information from many sources. The researcher is interested in

---

[1] The authors acknowledge the contributions of Karabenies et al. (1986) and Rowan (1981) in the development of these and subsequent lists of questions.

knowing if others perceive this as a problem and how they have dealt with it. *Thinking* involves more than a literature review, however; it is the use of data from any and all relevant sources: coworkers, or other women affected by the issue, for example, through interviews, telephone calls, word-of-mouth referrals. Here appears as well a historical phase in which the researcher investigates what has been done to identify emergent themes from actions taken in the past. It involves a dialogical encounter with people; instead of stating: "I have an idea," the researcher asks: "Here's an idea, what do you think of it? Where can we go with it?" (Duffy & Hedin, 1988, p. 534).

The *Thinking* phase involves the accumulation of information from many sources, combining and recombining it in new and creative ways. During this phase, the tension that exists originates in between the need for more information and the need to move on, to surpass what one has already found.

In feminist research, this phase involves intimate contact with women in identifying the problem, in identifying sources of information, and in their serving as resources for information. An effort is made to include women representing the study population as much as possible; client-advisory groups serve as one such workable means (Damrosch & Lenz, 1984).

Questions for Reflection during the Thinking Phase:

1. What are the chief concerns of the population that I am interested in working with?
2. How do they (the research participants) prioritize their research needs?
3. Does the literature reflect the experiences of the population?
4. How do women conceptualize the problem or need?
5. What are the various ways of stating the problem for this issue?
6. What is the history of the development of the conceptual framework?
7. Is the conceptual framework applicable to women, or does it reflect the male experience?
8. Is the historical significance of the problem under study fully developed, including its current status?

(Duffy & Hedin, 1988, p. 535)

The *Designing* Phase

Designing denotes that phase of researching in which a concrete plan is formulated from the many pieces of information gathered. The actual design of a feminist study takes women into account in the sampling, the relations within the research team, and specific attention to the everyday as a possible source of data, that is, day-to-day life as the starting point of research (Duffy & Hedin, 1988). During this phase, the tension that exists originates in that between the need to develop more plans, and the acceptance that enough plans have been generated. Participants are included in the planning whenever possible.

Questions for Reflection during the Designing Phase:

1. Are the opinions of each member of the research team solicited?
2. Is the discussion of research issues encouraged, or do I defend the "expert" position?
3. How can I encourage representatives of the study population to participate in all phases of the research?
4. Does the design of the study treat the participants as equals, or are they treated as objects used to collect data?
5. Does the design of the study investigate the societal and system-level factors that affect women?
6. Are the instruments used appropriate for the study of women?
7. Does the design allow for serendipitous findings, that is, the pursuit of intuitive clues?
8. Are my biases built into the study in any way?
9. Is the effect of context taken into account and allowed to express itself?
10. Are limitations imposed on who could be seen or on the types of questions asked? Do pressures to pursue a particular line of research exist?

(Duffy & Hedin, 1988, p. 535)

The *Encountering* Phase

It is during the *Encountering* phase that action, engagement, reflection, and reflection-in-action occur. During this phase the tension that exists originates in between perseverance and too much activity.

Questions for Reflection during the Encountering Phase:

1. Does the way I am carrying out the study make sense?
2. Am I open to my own feelings and reactions during the research process?

3. Am I communicating in a dialogical, nonhierarchical manner?

4. Am I breaking down control patterns?

5. Am I respecting the rights and dignity of colleagues and those participating in the study?

6. Am I doing any good? Any harm?

7. Am I expressing myself in an honest, authentic manner?

8. Am I following the experience where it naturally leads, but not to the detriment of study controls?

9. How are my values influencing the process?

(Duffy & Hedin, 1988, p. 537)

The *Making Sense* Phase

Making sense involves the analysis of and reflection on the data gathered. During this phase, the researcher attempts to move beyond unconscious presuppositions and assumptions to the discovery of the opaque and hidden meanings behind actions and spoken words. A deeper level of analysis is sought in which alternative ways of making sense of our world are found and created. Those structures and relations that have been found to oppress women are uncovered and exposed so that they can be transformed.

Whenever possible, the initial results are validated with the participants. There is an acknowledgement and living out of the belief that research is not an activity done alone, but in connectedness. The tension within this phase originates in the desire to reduce and simplify the data and the desire to make more and more connections so as to further clarify the results.

Questions for Reflection during the Making Sense Phase:

1. What are the participants' responses to the data?

2. Does my interpretation of the data make sense to the participants?

3. What alternative explanations exist for the data?

4. Are the findings politically useful for women?

5. Are the data compared to theories and standards that were developed for women and not the norms based on the experiences of men?

6. Does the analysis make biased assumptions—sexist, racist, or ageist?

7. Is the analysis liberating? Does it encourage others to raise questions?

(Duffy & Hedin, 1988, p. 537)

The *Communicating* Phase

Communicating is an outward movement—it meets the need to share what has occurred, but, in doing so, it encounters the tension that one cannot fully communicate with those who have not participated in the study. The researcher values sharing the results with the research participants; language is very important in doing this as well as the means chosen. The means may involve women's groups, lay magazines, individual mailings, and so forth. The intent of feminist research is that it is done *with* and *for* women and not *on* or *to* them (Duffy & Hedin, 1988).

Questions for Reflection during the Communicating Phase:

1. How can I reach the audience who represented the population of women participating in the study?
2. What language do I use to communicate the results?
3. For whom am I writing—women in general, or only the academic community?

(Duffy & Hedin, 1988, p. 538).

CONCLUSION

In this paper, we have discussed what it means to design research studies within a feminist perspective. In order to do this, a reconceptualization of the research process was described and envisioned as *Researching* with six phases: *Being, Thinking, Designing, Encountering, Making Sense,* and *Communicating.* The tensions that exist within each phase were described as well as the activities that occur. It is hoped that in this way the dynamic interplay that occurs within the process might be brought to the fore, and that the relationship between the means and ends of the research process might be highlighted. Cook and Fonow (1986) state that feminist methodology is in the process of becoming in the field of sociology; surely the same applies equally well to nursing. There is much yet to be explored, created, and envisioned as we open our minds to new paradigms.

REFERENCES

Bleier, R. (Ed.) (1986). *Feminist approaches to science*. New York: Pergamon Press.

Cook, J. A., & Fonow, M. M. (1986). Knowledge and women's interests: Issues of epistemology and methodology in feminist sociological research. *Sociological Inquiry, 56*(1), 2–29.

Damrosch, S. P., & Lenz, E. R. (1984). The use of client-advisory groups in research. *Nursing Research, 33*(1), 47–49.

Duffy, M. E. (1984). Transcending options: Creating a milieu for practicing high level wellness. *Health Care for Women International, 5*, 145–61.

Duffy, M. E., & Hedin, B. A. (1988). New directions for nursing research. In N. F. Woods & M. Catanzaro (Eds.), *Nursing research: Theory and practice* (pp. 530–39). St. Louis: C. V. Mosby.

Duffy, M. E., Mowbray, C., & Hudes, M. (1988). *The personal goals of recently divorced women: A feminist study*. Unpublished manuscript.

Fee, E. (1986). Critiques of modern science: The relationship of feminism to other radical epistemologies. In R. Bleier (Ed.), *Feminist approaches to science* (pp. 42–56). New York: Pergamon Press.

Harding, S. (1986). *The science question in feminism*. Ithaca, NY: Cornell University Press.

Hedin, B. A. (1986). A case study of oppressed group behavior in nurses. *Image, 18*(2), 53–57.

Hedin, B. A. (1987). Nursing education and social constraints: An in-depth analysis. *International Journal of Nursing Studies, 24*(3), 261–70.

Karabenies, A., Miller, L., Nagel-Bamesberger, H., Rossiter, A., & Thompson, M. (1986). What makes a feminist social science? *Cassandra: Radical Feminist Nurses Newsjournal, 4*(1), 9–11.

MacPherson, K. I. (1983). Feminist methods: A new paradigm for nursing research. *Advances in Nursing Science, 5*(2), 17–25.

Namenwirth, M. (1986). Science seen through a feminist prism. In R. Bleier (Ed.), *Feminist approaches to science* (pp. 18–41). New York: Pergamon Press.

Rose, H. (1986). Beyond masculinist realities: A feminist epistemology for the sciences. In R. Bleier (Ed.), *Feminist approaches to science* (pp. 57–76). New York: Pergamon Press.

Rowan, J. (1981). A dialectical paradigm for research. In P. Reason & J. Rowan (Eds.), *Human inquiry: A sourcebook of new paradigm research*. New York: John Wiley.

Stanley, L., & Wise, S. (1983). *Breaking out: Feminist consciousness and feminist research*. London: Routledge & Kegan Paul.